Running on Veggies

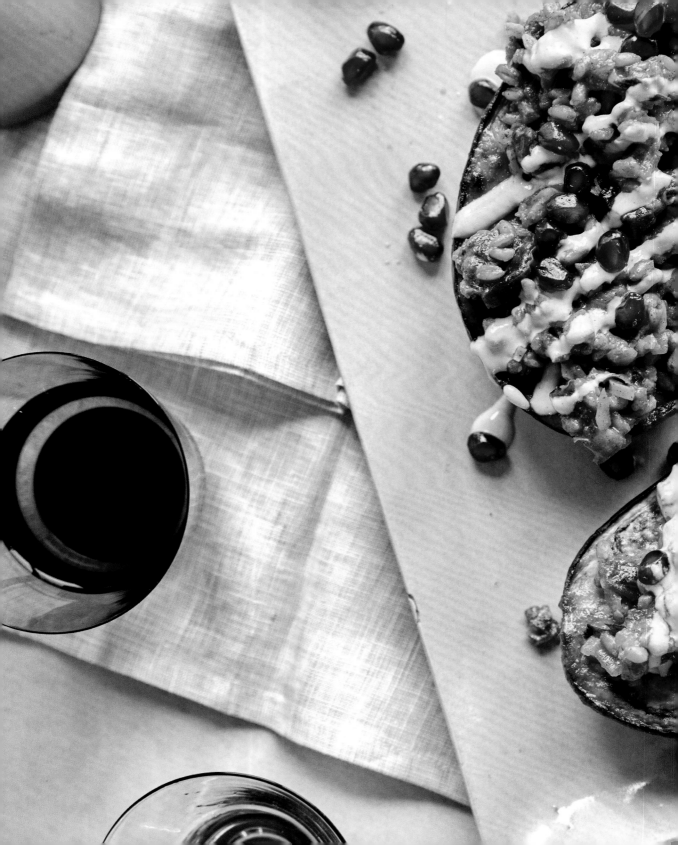

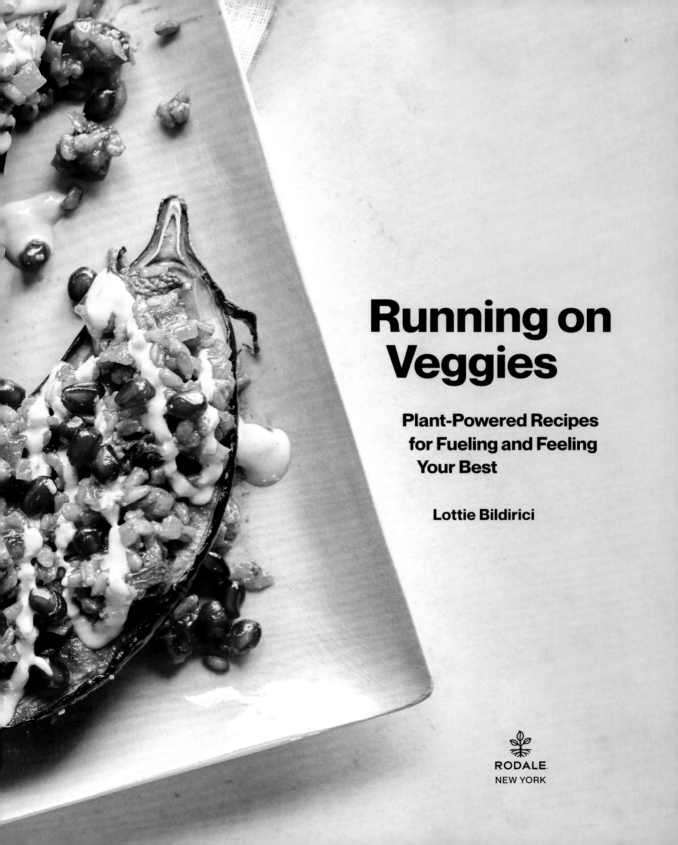

Running on Veggies

Plant-Powered Recipes for Fueling and Feeling Your Best

Lottie Bildirici

RODALE

NEW YORK

Photographs by Keith Montero on pages 4, 5, 11 (right), 15, 19,
246, 248, and 249. Photograph by Susan Menashe on page 11
(left). Photographs by Donalrey Nieva on pages 12, 13, and 181.
Illustrations by Emily Sundberg on pages 23 and 33.

Library of Congress Cataloging-in-Publication Data
Names: Bildirici, Lottie, author.
Title: Running on veggies : plant-powered recipes for fueling
    and feeling your best / Lottie Bildirici.
Description: New York : Rodale, [2021] | Includes index.
Identifiers: LCCN 2021004232 (print) | LCCN 2021004233
    (ebook) | ISBN 9780593231715 (hardcover) | ISBN
    9780593231722 (ebook)
Subjects: LCSH: Vegetarian cooking. | Cooking (Vegetables) |
    LCGFT: Cookbooks.
Classification: LCC TX837 .B525 2021 (print) | LCC TX837
    (ebook) | DDC 641.5/636--dc23
LC record available at https://lccn.loc.gov/2021004232
LC ebook record available at https://lccn.loc.gov
    /2021004233

ISBN 978-0-593-23171-5
Ebook ISBN 978-0-593-23172-2

Printed in China

Book design by Jennifer K. Beal Davis and Lise Sukhu
Jacket design by Jennifer K. Beal Davis
Jacket photographs by Lauren Volo

Photographer: Lauren Volo
Food stylist: Monica Pierini
Food stylist assistant: Emma Rowe
Prop stylist: Maeve Sheridan
Editor: Dervla Kelly
Designers: Jennifer K. Beal Davis and Lise Sukhu
Production editor: Joyce Wong
Production manager: Philip Leung
Composition: Merri Ann Morrell and Hannah Hunt
Copy editor: Jude Grant
Indexer: Elizabeth T. Parson

10 9 8 7 6 5 4 3 2 1

First Edition

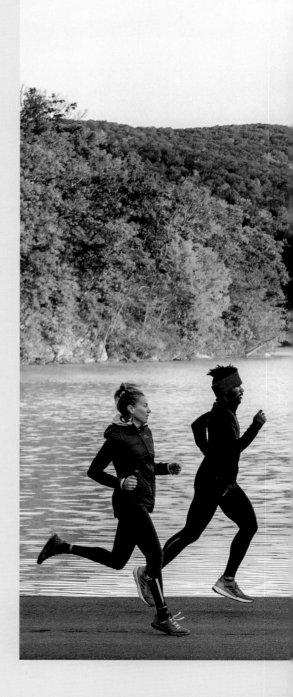

This book is dedicated to my mother and my grandma, Lottie, whose doors were always open and whose tables were always set. I hope that my kitchen is as warm and inviting as hers has always been to our family and community.

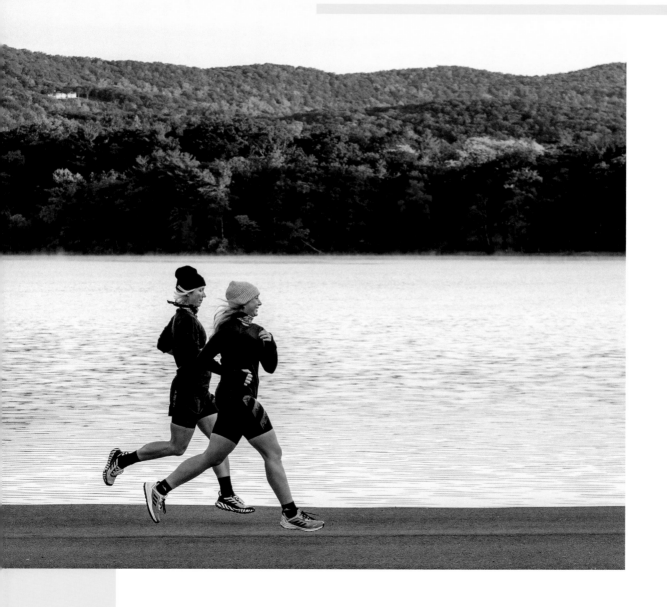

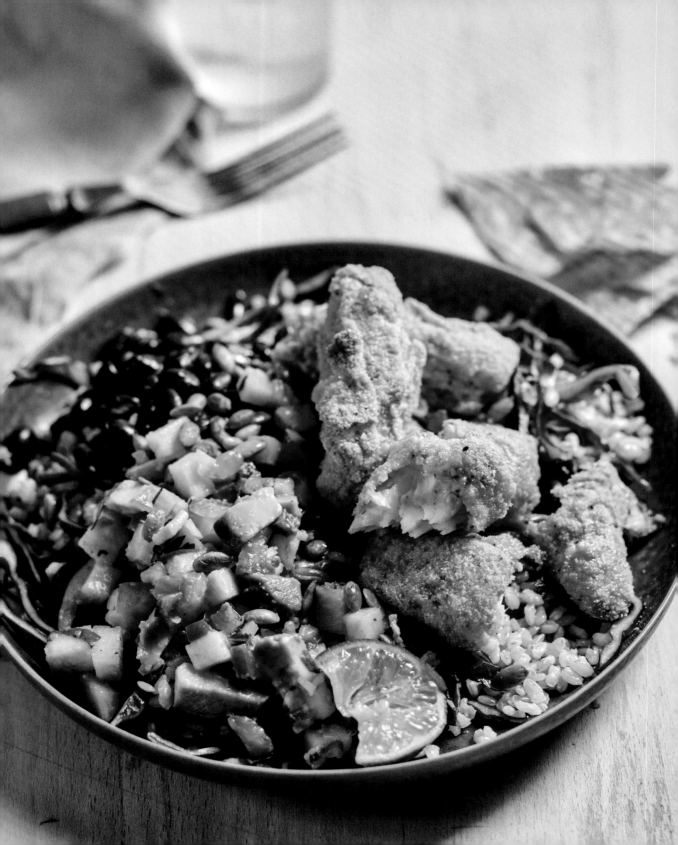

Contents

My Story

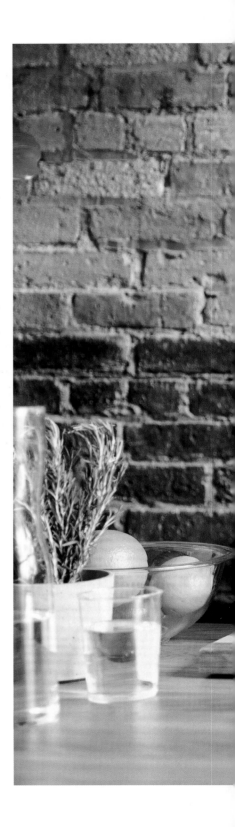

My earliest childhood memories take place in the kitchen. It was the central hub of my home, and it was where I often joined my mother and grandmother, who seemed to be perpetually immersed in cooking and conversation. My family is famous for its legacy of preparing, cooking, and serving others. This legacy has been passed down from generation to generation.

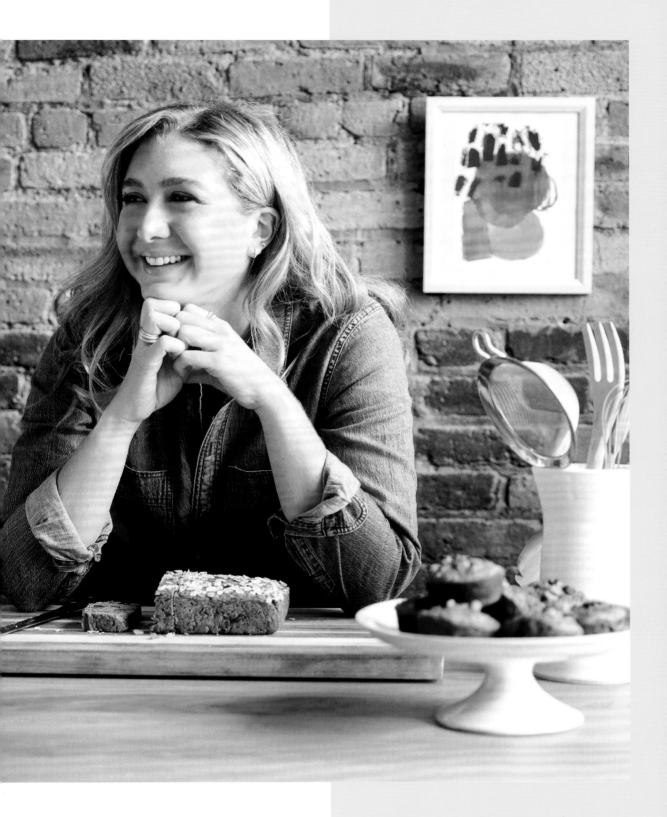

I grew up listening to tales of my grandmother Lottie. It is tradition in my family to name your children after your parents. My grandmother was not fond of her name and convinced my mother's sisters not to name their daughters after her. But my mom stuck to tradition, and although I have a handful of female cousins, I'm the only Lottie. I love being her namesake, and I think the fact that I'm the only other Lottie is no accident. I'm fairly certain I inherited more than her name. She was known for feeding the mailman every day when he delivered mail, and she would show up to her doctors' appointments with fresh baked blueberry muffins. My journey toward making health, fitness, and nutrition my life's work didn't begin with that legacy, however.

In 2008, when I was fourteen years old, I was diagnosed with Stage III Hodgkin's Lymphoma. I was a freshman in high school with few cares beyond friends, relationships, homework, and hobbies. The day was routine, like every other before it. I reached my hand up to remove my necklace when I noticed a bump on my neck. My parents' immediate alarm scared me, and it wasn't long before we found ourselves in front of the doctor who dropped the news into our laps: I had cancer. And in that moment, I went from high school freshman to cancer patient.

I knew the hospital hallways like the back of my hands: the vending machines, that one ugly painting they refused to take down, the room where they'd pump me full of chemo. My skin hollowed, my hair fell out. Eyebrows. Eyelashes. I felt like I was losing my identity. I wish I could say the nausea was the worst of it, but it was only a small part. Like all teenagers, I was desperate to fit in. But I couldn't. My new normal was me trying to forget the alienating feeling of being sick and different in a world where conformity is king. By tenth grade, I had successfully pushed aside the psychological pain, wrapped it up, and locked it in a box in the attic of my mind so it couldn't hurt me anymore—or so I thought.

I had succeeded (for the most part) in ignoring those painful months, but senior year of high school brought those memories back to light.

A group of people from my neighborhood were going to Disney World to run a half-marathon and raise money for a community cancer center that had helped my family and me when I was going through treatment. It was the perfect opportunity to give back and also to give myself permission to speak a bit more openly about my experience. I had never run before, although I had always been athletic. I didn't even know what it meant to run a 5K. As I did with all things in my life, I jumped in headfirst and put my all into the training. If I was going to do this race, I wanted to be prepared. After a few months of training, I showed up to that start line overflowing with emotions. I was a survivor, a warrior, a giver . . . and now, a runner. My story seemed to come full circle in that moment, and I finally felt healed—body and soul. Running that race was the first time I felt in control of my life again. On that starting line, I felt powerful, in control of my life, like I hadn't before cancer. It was a jumping-off point.

After that race, I began to do some real thinking about what was going on in my body. Did I eat the right thing before the race? Was there a way to shave time off my best? Could I make a small change that might help me recover more quickly?

Unlike my battle with cancer, this was something I could control. I could control my input and output, make sure my body was getting what it needed, and account for every nutritional deficit. After being pumped full of drugs and heavy chemotherapy treatments, I felt like my body needed a reset.

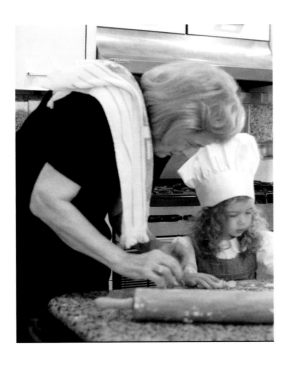
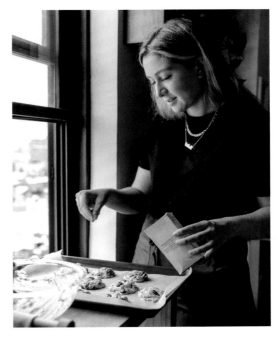

I fell in love with athletic competition after Disney and went on to compete in multiple distance races. I got faster and faster, breathed better, reveled in the burn of muscle and the sharp exhales on otherwise quiet trails. Having researched food heavily and realizing its importance, I started creating healthier diets for myself. There were "healthy" foods and "unhealthy" foods. But it wasn't just enough to limit or portion control the unhealthy foods—I had to eliminate them altogether.

You may know where this is going, but I sure didn't at the time. Soon enough, it wasn't just about eliminating those "unhealthy" foods but a genuine fear I developed when it came to those foods. I became food obsessed, a slave to my own phobia, terrified of upsetting the perfect utopia palace that was my body, my temple. I lost sight of the larger picture. I pored over ingredients, assessed macros, measured my servings, and weighed my portions. I barely blinked when my period stopped; hey, if all the best serious athletes also stopped menstruating, didn't that mean I was a serious athlete too? The purer I became, the more my body deteriorated. Eventually, as a lifesaving measure, my body chose to rebel.

Looking back, what strikes me is not that I injured myself but that I was more upset about not being able to run than the seemingly spontaneous breakage of my body.

I was angry, frustrated, and disappointed. In trying to take control of my body after cancer, I had stepped over the psychological line between health consciousness and an eating disorder. My daily functioning had been taken over by the obsession and I found myself losing control once

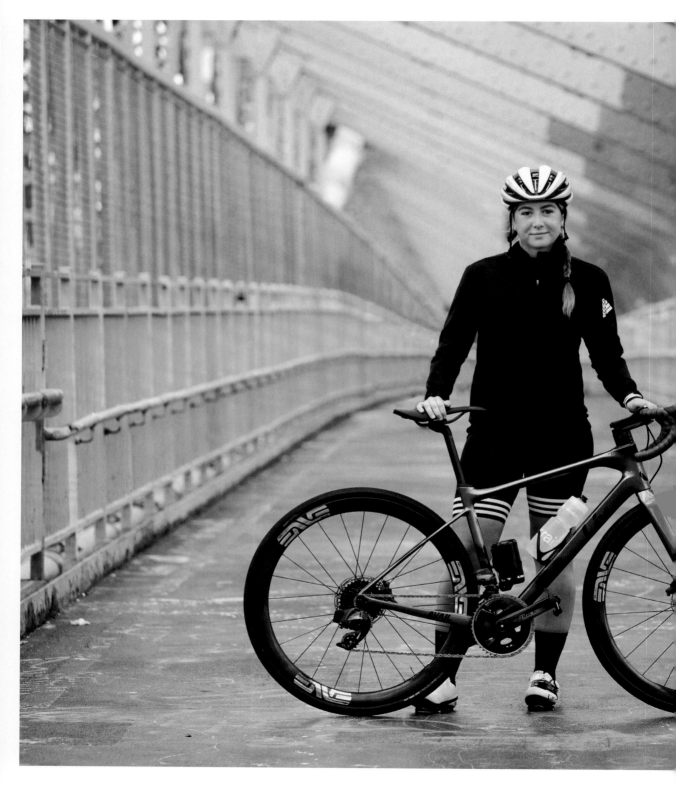

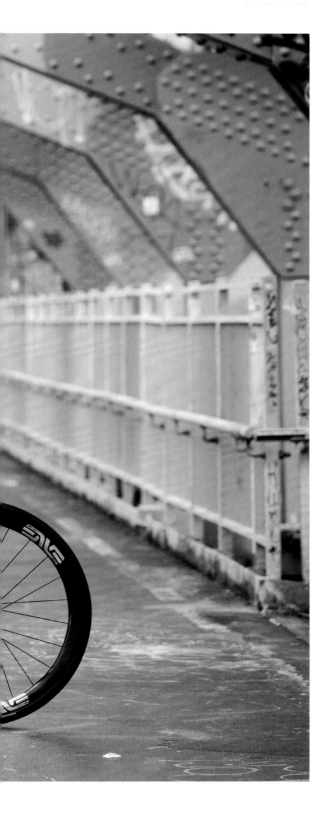

more. After my fourth stress fracture in four years, I finally realized that I needed to make a decided effort to reverse my so-called health obsession and begin my healing anew.

It took significant effort, but I soon began to associate food not as healthy and unhealthy options but rather as fuel. Restrictive eating became intuitive eating. The journey was not by any means easy—I suffered a few setbacks—but my recovery was steady and inevitable. As during that first race, I was determined to make it to the other side, emerge with a healthy body and mind.

Unfortunately, amenorrhea, eating disorders, and pathological relationships with food are all too common among female athletes. Throughout my own journey, I had connected with many people and found community within our struggles and triumphs. Education and support were critical for me, and I wanted to create a platform where the mutual learning and encouragement could continue.

That's how *Running on Veggies* was born. It represented a shared mission: healing through food, running stronger, cycling faster, and preventing injury. I belonged.

I have helped some of the best athletes in the world achieve their nutritional and athletic goals in the last decade. I even began sharing my cancer story—one I'd been so adamant in hiding and locking away in my effort to fit in and return to normalcy. Cancer happened to me; it didn't define me. Looking back, I really wish I'd had a role model when my world was shattered, one who faced adversity head-on, who exemplified courage and strength, who wasn't afraid to own their story. That's why on the ten-year anniversary of my diagnosis, I competed in an Ironman triathlon— 2.4-mile swim, 112-mile bike, and 26.2-mile run—not just to prove to myself and others I could do it but also as a platform to share my story openly and proudly.

My Ironman training helped solidify my theory of food as fuel, and I learned (through trial and error) how I could satisfy and propel my body forward efficiently. It was as much a nutrition game as it was an endurance challenge. I focused on recovery, making sure I was fueling with foods that would allow me to be ready for the next day's workout. Working full time and training for an Ironman was intense. I was up before dawn most days, but I managed to take good care of myself. I didn't always get a full eight hours of sleep in, but nothing could stop me from tackling this challenge. I learned I had to choose myself day after day, and part of my growth and healing was proving to myself that I could accomplish amazing things while being smart about my dietary choices.

After months of training and juggling an overwhelming schedule, the day of the triathlon finally arrived. Yes, my feet were tired and my muscles were screaming, but above all I felt an overwhelming sense of relief and pride—pride that my body was healthy and strong enough to keep going, put one foot in front of the other, push myself that much further. I finished and earned a spot in the Ironman World Championship in Kona, but ultimately I realized I had another calling. Although I still enjoy distance running, long bike rides, and a casual 5:00 a.m. swim, I wanted to focus on giving back. I wanted to inspire others to recognize the strength in themselves, to admire the beauty of strength and stamina. That is why I wrote this book.

Career

Growing up in an insular community and traditional household in Brooklyn, I was not expected to pursue higher education or a professional career. I may have continued on that path if not for my battle with cancer. I started asking questions, like "Why not?" "Why can't I?" and "If not now, when?" I figured if I could come out successful against an uphill battle with cancer, how hard could a few gender norms be? Out of this adversity, an indefatigable work ethic had emerged.

At seventeen, I started my own business selling healthy desserts from my mother's kitchen. My mother hated when I made a mess in her kitchen, but somehow I always found my way back in. I sold vegan cakes, raw truffles, and cookies—I played around with all kinds of ingredients and experimented with different baking techniques.

I was my most creative when I crafted new recipes, put my own spin on a popular dessert, or switched ingredients around to the delight of my friends and family. It may seem small in the grand scheme of things, but working in Mother's kitchen gave me the confidence to think about a career in the food space, although it would be a while before I saw food creation as a lucrative career. I learned how powerful word of mouth was, and my success skyrocketed; I was baking all weekend, in between homework, and alongside applying for colleges.

At college, I continued on with my life, still baking in between 5:00 a.m. runs, classes, and even a coveted internship in the music industry. The only part I enjoyed was the early morning runs, but to be honest, the adrenaline rush didn't really make the rest of the day any more satisfying.

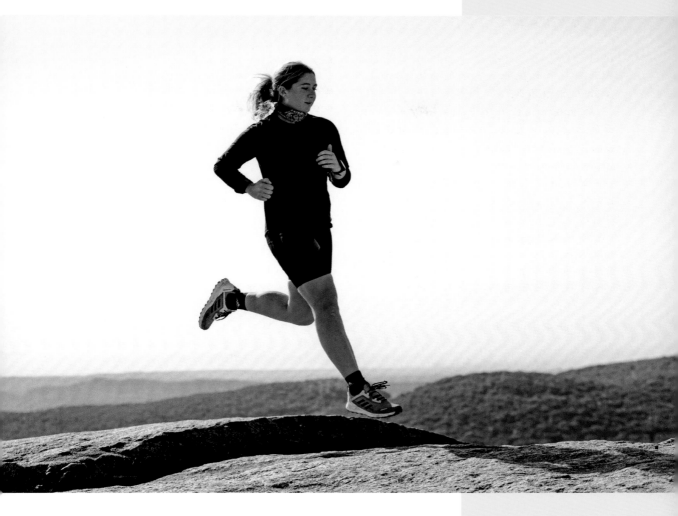
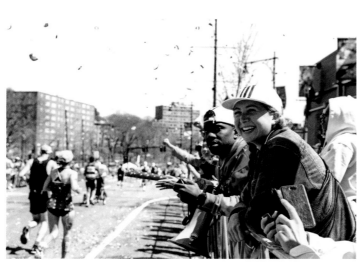

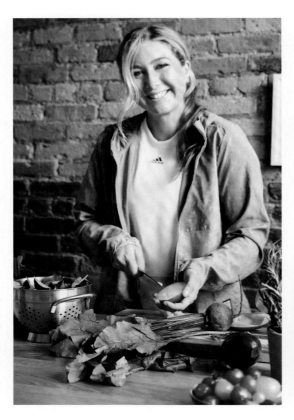

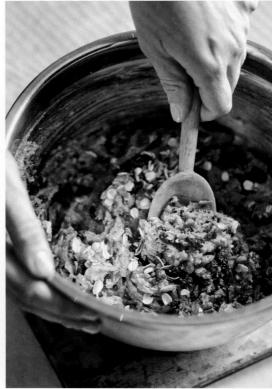

One day, I was sitting at my office with the tray of vegan soft-baked cookies I had brought for my coworkers, and as they were happily munching and complimenting me on my baking, it hit me: the adrenaline rush I was chasing was not running but making people feel good through food! Watching people in my office stop by my desk for a cookie (or two . . . or three) was more fulfilling than any of my internship work. I realized in that moment that I could never have a standard desk job.

I hit the ground running (no pun intended) and started my Running on Veggies journey. After two years of managing my blog and social media, I had acquired a small but meaningful community of followers. It was around that time when Kara

Goucher, a well-known distance runner and one of my personal idols, reached out to me to speak at her upcoming running retreat in Napa, California. She had found me on social media and enjoyed the approachable way in which I discussed nutrition and recipes. I was shocked and a bit star struck! An amazing person like her seeking my advice? I realized I had a captivated audience of experienced runners who were genuinely interested in what I had to say. The sense of belonging to a community propelled me forward yet again. I said yes to Kara and got to work.

In 2015, Kara was hosting another retreat, this time in Breckenridge, Colorado, and she invited me to come a week early and stay with her in

Boulder, where she lives and trains. While I was there, I decided to cook a bit for her. Her coaches noticed that after just a week of eating my meals, snacks, and desserts, she was training harder and recovering faster.

I felt so validated in my beliefs about food when her coaches suggested Kara have me return to Boulder and stay with her to help her train for the marathon Olympic trials. If she could make it to the top three, this would be her second time on the US marathon team. I hightailed back to New York to pack my things and then headed to Boulder for the entire winter. I made sure Kara ate the necessary fuel for her workouts until the trials, and the progress she made in training was inspiring.

February 2016 found us in Los Angeles for the trials. The temperature on race day was in the mid-90s, but Kara ran hard, passing almost everyone in the latter part of the race and placing fourth, just one spot shy of the Olympic team. Although she didn't place in the top three, the results from my diet plan on her performance could not be overstated.

What I didn't realize at the time was that quite a few elite athletes were following my work with Kara. That attention led to opportunities for me to work with Olympians, World Champions, professional cycling teams, and even runner Stephanie Bruce, who was training for the same Olympic trials race that Kara had competed in four years earlier.

I continued to pursue my career in helping athletes leverage nutrition to perform at peak levels. More important, I also continued to focus on making my knowledge and recipes accessible for my followers online. My recipes were being picked up by various publications and websites, and I was featured on morning talk shows and a magazine cover.

In 2018, I joined Adidas as the North American Nutrition Coach for the Adidas Runners community. Adidas Runners is a global running community built on a holistic framework, so I get to work alongside coaches to assist everyday athletes in their weekly training programs.

The opportunity to work with both professional and everyday athletes and share my experiences and knowledge about the body and mind relationship to food with my public following is a dream come true. I fought against insurmountable odds and succeeded, and now I have the opportunity to share my journey with you all. Thank you for your love and support. Bon appétit!

Food Philosophy

I have experienced firsthand how integral food is to health and well-being. You'll find my approach to cooking and eating is simple—keep it real! I've found that the best daily diet comprises nutrient-dense whole foods with few ingredients and lots of vegetables. Processed foods and foods with added sugars, preservatives, or chemicals are not foods that will "work for us" as they are digested. By this, I mean they will not contribute much to your health or optimal performance. That's not to say all processed foods are necessarily bad for you. "Healthy" and "unhealthy" food categories are not what I'm about. But if you want your food to make your body stronger and healthier (and I think most of us do!), the whole foods approach is the way to go.

And while this is certainly the optimal choice across the board, the actual balance of foods, macros, and vitamins that each individual needs will vary from person to person depending on the circumstances. It is important not to label your diet, as that will set up the potential for straying

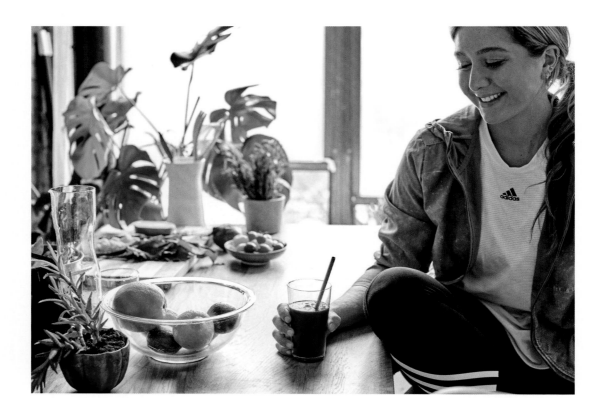

from your plan. Your diet should be fluid and ever changing, just as hormones, age, environment, health, and goals are ever changing.

The recipes in this book reflect my own personal healthy-eating habits and were crafted with tastes, textures, and ingredients that I think you'll enjoy as much as I do. However, these recipes are meant to be flexible and personalized. For example, while I don't eat red meat, someone who does might choose to use meat instead of fish in my Homemade BBQ Salmon (page 125). I hope you'll feel comfortable playing with the recipes and trying out what combinations work for you.

I have also crafted all my recipes using natural sweeteners. I believe food can be tasty without all those artificial sweeteners and chemicals, and I want to show you how. If you focus on whole foods, then you'll inevitably stay away from these types of sweeteners. That being said, a number of recipes in this book call for maple syrup, which I have found to be the most nutrient dense and most innocuous of all the many sugar additives. It is rich in magnesium, zinc, and calcium and works well in the "adventure snacks," which are meant to be eaten during endurance workouts. Maple syrup is the perfect antidote to restocking all the energy that your body burns during long

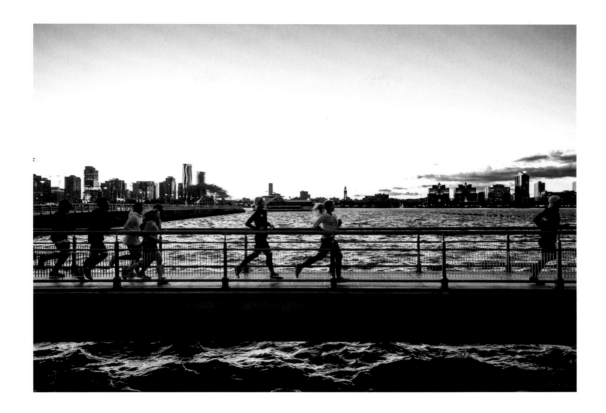

rides, runs, and hikes. I also use maple syrup in my dessert recipes because we all need an occasional treat or indulgence every now and then.

Along with keeping it real, I also believe in keeping it simple. A healthy diet does not have to necessitate tons of time and effort. I know from years of health coaching that if cooking a certain way is too complicated, it just won't get done. Because we need to fuel ourselves multiple times a day, every single day, cooking needs to be something we can do easily and quickly without compromising health standards. Since our bodies are the best indicator of whether or not our food

is working for us, I don't offer calorie counts or macro breakdowns of my recipes. Instead, pay attention to your energy level, comfort level, and satiety. If you experience warning signs such as chronic fatigue, headaches, bloating, or any other discomforts, these are signals that something needs to change in your diet. Tune in to your body before and after you eat so that you become practiced at reading its cues. It is this intuitive eating philosophy that has helped my clients of all levels break barriers in their own performances and fitness.

The
Pantry

Keeping a well-stocked pantry with the right ingredients is essential to making recipes efficiently and quickly. And it also helps you make the right choices. Here are some of the ingredients that I make sure are in my kitchen every week.

Dry Savory Goods

- **Organic canned goods:** I tend to buy canned beans and tomatoes since it saves a lot of time during busy weeks. I look for organic canned goods that are salt-free. My favorite items are chickpeas, black beans, cannellini beans, and crushed tomatoes.

- **Low-sodium vegetable stock:** Feel free to use water if you don't have stock, but veggie stock adds so much more flavor. I like using low sodium so you can control the salt amount yourself.

- **Unsweetened full-fat and light coconut milk:** When I'm looking to add creaminess to a dish, I add a little bit of coconut milk and it usually does the trick. It also adds vitamins and minerals like vitamins C, E, and B_1 plus iron, calcium, and phosphorous.

- **Tomato paste:** If you want to take a tomato-based recipe or a recipe with a strong tomato presence up a flavor notch, add a tablespoon or two of tomato paste. Be sure to cook the paste a minute or so to allow the natural sugars to caramelize.

- **Lentils:** These legumes are a great source of protein and cook quickly compared to others. Lentils provide fiber, iron, folic acid, and magnesium.

- **Brown rice, wild rice, and white rice:** Rice is great for veggie bowls and is a good addition to soups and stews. My day-to-day go-to is brown or wild rice, but I do eat white rice during workouts or intense training periods when I'm burning a lot of energy since it's easier to digest.

- **Whole grains:** I keep several different types of whole grains, like quinoa and farro, in my pantry at all times. They are full of vitamins and also are a good source of protein. They are perfect to add to a salad or use instead of rice in a vegetable bowl.

- **Whole grain or plant-based pastas:** My main pasta go-tos are brown rice pasta and chickpea pasta. They are both perfect for a quick red sauce or pesto on a weeknight.

- **Nuts:** Nuts are something I buy in bulk and store in the freezer, so they don't spoil too quickly. I always have almonds, cashews, pecans, and walnuts on hand, and I buy them raw so that I can toast them and add salt or spices while I'm cooking.

- **Seeds:** Seeds add a crunch to any recipe, savory or sweet, as well as a nutty, rich flavor. I love using sesame seeds, pumpkin seeds (pepitas), sunflower seeds, and chia seeds.

- **Plant-based protein powders:** These are great to have around for smoothies as well as baked goods. I look for non-GMO plant-based protein powders that are unsweetened or stevia sweetened. Be sure to also look for a protein powder that has at least 15 grams of protein per serving. I often buy unflavored, but vanilla and chocolate are delicious too. If you are using vanilla and chocolate, you don't need vanilla extract and you can reduce the cocoa powder in a recipe to your liking.

Baking

- **Gluten-free flours:** The main gluten-free flours I use in this book are oat flour and almond flour since they are the most accessible. But of course feel free to experiment with your favorite gluten-free flours.

- **White whole wheat flour:** This is the same as regular whole wheat flour except it's milled from a white wheatberry rather than a red wheatberry. I like using white whole wheat flour for its mild flavor as well as the superior texture it gives to dense baked goods, like quick breads and some cakes.

- **Oats:** There are three types of oats: steel-cut oats, old-fashioned rolled oats, and quick-cooking oats. All three of these oats go through the initial process of having the inedible hull removed from the whole oat kernel.

  - **Steel-cut oats:** Steel-cut oats are the least processed form of oats and also take the longest to cook. They have a chewy, nutty flavor. I like using them for oat bowls or savory recipes.

  - **Old-fashioned rolled oats:** When I'm adding oats to a baked good, these are the ones I opt for. They have gone through a steaming and rolling process that doesn't significantly affect their health benefits, and they have a milder flavor than steel-cut oats and give great tender texture to baked goods.

  - **Quick-cooking oats:** I stay away from quick-cooking oats, which includes instant oats. These oats are the most processed and go through an additional steaming and rolling process that makes them even thinner and more pre-cooked than rolled oats. They have the quickest cooking time as a result, but a mushy texture. Since they are more broken down than steel-cut or old-fashioned oats, they don't keep you feeling full as long.

- **Coconut oil:** I always use cold-pressed, unrefined virgin coconut oil. It's the least processed of all the coconut oils and also has the richest flavor. I use coconut oil in baking because of its mild flavor, which pairs nicely with sweet flavors and warm spices.

- **Medjool dates:** Dates are my main sweetener when it comes to anything savory or sweet. I like to sweeten my recipes with fruit rather than refined sugars. By using the whole date, you are adding additional fiber as well as vitamins and minerals like iron, potassium, and copper to a recipe.

- **Pure maple syrup:** Syrup is an ingredient I use only in my adventure snacks and desserts. It provides a little extra sweetness and maple flavor when compared to dates. Maple syrup also has some health benefits: it contains antioxidants and small amounts of manganese and zinc, both beneficial minerals. It also has a lower glycemic index than granulated sugar. If you can find Grade B maple, try it—it has a richer, deeper flavor and is higher in antioxidants than the lighter Grade A.

- **Coconut sugar and date sugar:** These two sugars are sweeteners I use only in desserts when a recipe, like cookies, just needs that classic sugar texture.

  - **Coconut sugar:** This is made from the coconut palm sap, which is the sugary liquid from the coconut plant. The liquid sap of the coconut palm or coconut tree is boiled until most of the water has evaporated and sugar is left, which is the sugary liquid from the flower buds of the coconut tree. Coconut sugar contains small amounts of minerals like iron, zinc, calcium, and potassium. It also has

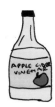
APPLE CIDER VINEGAR

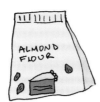
ALMOND FLOUR

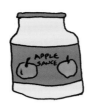
APPLE SAUCE

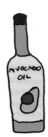
AVOCADO OIL

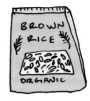
BROWN RICE
ORGANIC

CAULIFLOWER RICE

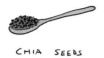
CHIA SEEDS

COCONUT

COCONUT OIL

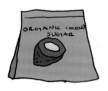
ORGANIC COCONUT SUGAR

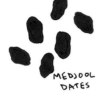
MEDJOOL DATES

FLAX SEEDS organic

FROZEN PEAS

FROZEN SPINACH

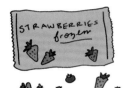
STRAWBERRIES frozen

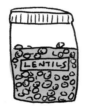
LENTILS

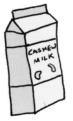
CASHEW MILK

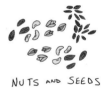
NUTS AND SEEDS

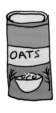
OATS

Whole grain Pasta

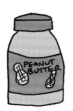
PEANUT BUTTER

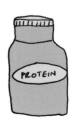
PROTEIN

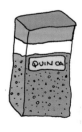
QUINOA

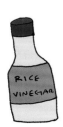
RICE VINEGAR

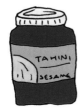
TAHINI SESAME

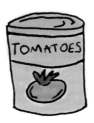
TOMATOES

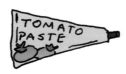
TOMATO PASTE

STOCK

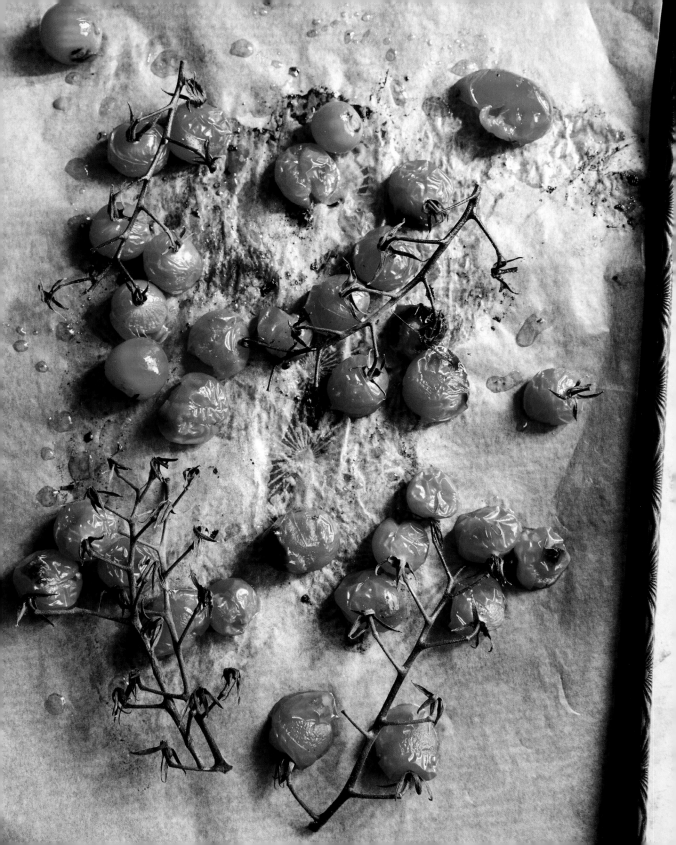

a fiber called inulin, which may contribute to it having a slightly lower glycemic index than granulated sugar.

- **Date sugar:** This is slightly different since it's made from dried dates. As a result of using the whole fruit, date sugar has the fiber, nutrients, vitamins, minerals, and antioxidants that are found in whole dates. It also has a lower glycemic index than granulated sugar. It isn't as sweet as regular sugar when used in baked goods but gives a nice caramel-like flavor that's still delicious.

- **Unsweetened applesauce:** Applesauce is an alternative binder to egg and also adds moisture to a baked good. I always have some unsweetened applesauce in the cupboard in case I want to substitute an egg in a recipe.

- **Unsweetened nut milk:** I often use any unsweetened nut milk as the dairy-free liquid binder for a recipe. Its mild flavor and lightly rich texture help make a chocolate cake that much more decadent than using only water. Nut milk is a little sweeter than regular milk and can be lighter in texture depending on how much fat content is in the regular milk you buy.

- **Unsweetened full-fat or light coconut milk:** I turn to coconut milk in desserts that need a thicker and creamier milk than a nut milk, like certain cakes, creamy pie fillings, and puddings. Coconut milk is also the key to making dairy-free ice cream and is the main ingredient in my ice cream cake recipes (see page 224–25). Be sure to shake the coconut milk well before using.

- **Ground flaxseed:** Not only is flax rich in omega-3s and fiber, ground flaxseed also acts as a great binding agent in baked goods. For a good egg substitute, use 1 tablespoon ground flaxseed to 2 to 3 tablespoons water. Allow to thicken for 5 to 10 minutes. Be sure to buy ground flaxseed since it's much easier for the body to digest than whole flaxseed.

- **Chia seeds:** Chia seeds are great in baking because they absorb liquid well, helping bind baked goods and give them moisture. I like to use them in cakes and quick breads in place of eggs. They also boast a ton of nutritional qualities, like being a great source of omega-3s, fiber, iron, and calcium. In place of 1 egg, use 1 tablespoon of chia seeds mixed with 3 tablespoons of water. Allow to sit for 5 minutes, then use.

- **Unsweetened natural nut butters:** Nut butters can add a delicious, rich flavor to any baked good. They are a great source of healthy fats and work as a binder in baking recipes. Be sure to look for natural and unsweetened varieties when choosing nut butters. The only ingredient should be nuts.

- **Unsweetened cocoa powder:** This ingredient is key for anything chocolate. I use unsweetened cocoa powder since it has none of the added sugars that many bar chocolates contain. Cocoa powder is rich in polyphenols, which are natural antioxidants. The antioxidants found in cocoa powder have been shown to help reduce inflammation, lower blood pressure, and improve cholesterol levels.

- **Dark chocolate chips:** I look for stevia-sweetened vegan dark chocolate chips, such as Lily's, to avoid added sugar when I just want chocolate in a recipe. They are so delicious and give you all that cravable chocolate flavor.

Oils, Vinegars, and Spices

- **Avocado oil:** When it comes to cooking anything savory with high temperature, unrefined avocado oil is my preference. It's a heart-healthy fat with a higher smoke point than olive oil, perfect for the stovetop.

- **Extra-virgin olive oil:** *Extra-virgin* means the oil was extracted through cold pressing. It's also a heart-healthy oil and has been shown to lower the risk of certain cancers and improve cholesterol. I use olive oil for uncooked savory foods like salad dressings and hummus, and I'll drizzle it on top of toast or a stew to finish the dish before serving. Be sure to look at the label and make sure it is a pure extra-virgin olive oil and not an olive oil blend.

- **Tahini:** This sesame seed paste is full of so many healthy fats and adds a rich, nutty flavor to any savory or sweet recipe. It's also one of the richest sources of plant-based calcium and iron. I like to add a spoonful of tahini to a salad dressing, smoothie, roasted vegetables, and even some dessert recipes.

- **Apple cider vinegar:** I'm a fan of any vinegar, but apple cider is my favorite since it has so many health benefits. I try to buy unfiltered apple cider vinegar with the "mother," which has proteins, enzymes, and good bacteria for the gut.

- **Unseasoned rice wine vinegar:** I love using rice wine vinegar for its light acidic / slightly sweet taste. It's perfect for pickling and using in salad dressings. This vinegar is made from fermented rice and is known to help with digestive health and reduce inflammation.

- **Balsamic vinegar:** Balsamic is the vinegar I use to add flavor to a dish needing "something else," like a marinade or dressing. It's bolder in taste than apple cider and rice vinegar. Balsamic has also been found to regulate blood sugar after eating and help with digestive health.

- **Spices:** I love using chili powder, cumin, ground coriander, cinnamon, sweet paprika, smoked paprika, red chili flakes, and oregano. Refer to Flavor Guide (opposite page) for additional ideas for using spices.

Frozen Foods

- **Fruit:** I always have three or four different types of frozen fruit for smoothies or desserts in my freezer. Be sure to peel and freeze any overripe bananas. They are perfect for smoothies.

- **Cauliflower rice:** This is the perfect freezer staple that lasts a long time and goes with almost any meal. Whenever I need a base to a bowl recipe or a side dish, I sauté some cauliflower rice with spices and other veggies.

- **Frozen greens:** Keeping greens in the freezer is an easy way to add vitamins and nutrients to smoothies or savory recipes, like a stew, right before serving. Kale and spinach are my preferred frozen greens.

- **Peas and corn:** Peas and corn are two veggies I like to add a handful of to a soup, sauce, or pasta recipe. They add quick vegetable flavor and nutrients.

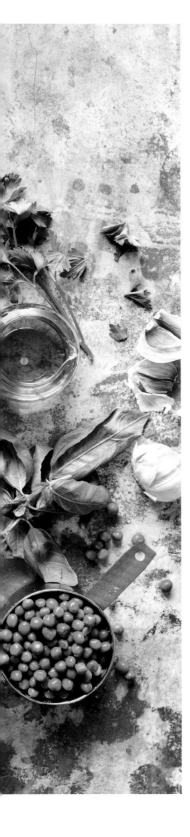

Flavor Guide

When I'm coming up with a new recipe, I find this Flavor Guide very helpful as a reference for some of the common spices and ingredients used in different cuisines. Try using it yourself to make the simplest of recipes rich in taste.

Chinese flavors

Fresh ginger
Garlic
Scallions
Fresh cilantro
Limes
Toasted sesame oil
Rice wine vinegar
Unsweetened chili sauce or red chili flakes
Miso paste
Liquid aminos (I like Bragg)
Water chestnuts
Peanuts
Sesame seeds

Italian flavors

Oregano, dried or fresh
Rosemary, dried or fresh
Fresh flat-leaf parsley
Fresh basil
Garlic
Fresh fennel or dried fennel seed
Red chili flakes
Tomato paste
Red wine vinegar
Balsamic vinegar
Nutritional yeast

Thai flavors

Thai curry paste
Fresh ginger
Garlic
Scallions
Lemongrass
Fresh basil or Thai basil
Fresh cilantro
Fresh mint
Limes
Sriracha
Coconut milk
Peanuts

Mexican flavors

Cayenne pepper or hot sauce
Chili powder
Ground cumin or cumin seed
Ground cinnamon
Mexican dried oregano
Unsweetened cocoa powder
Oranges
Limes and lemons
Fresh cilantro
Jalapeño or serrano

Mediterranean flavors

Lemons
Fresh mint
Fresh flat-leaf parsley
Oregano, dried or fresh
Fresh dill
Ground coriander or coriander seed
Ground cumin or cumin seed
Paprika
Ground turmeric
Red wine vinegar
Balsamic vinegar
Tahini

Indian flavors

Garlic
Fresh ginger
Fresh cilantro
Curry powder
Garam masala
Ground cumin or cumin seed
Ground fennel or fennel seed
Star anise
Ground turmeric or fresh turmeric root
Cardamom pods or ground cardamom
Coconut milk

Equipment List

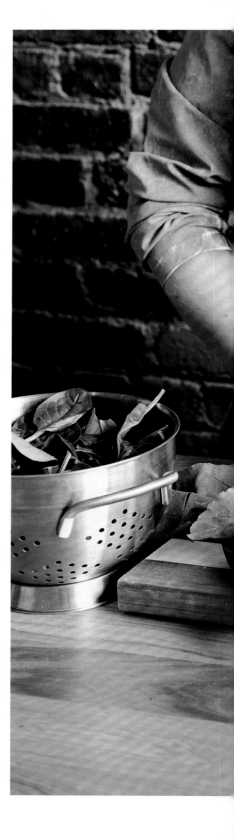

- 9 × 5-inch loaf pan
- Muffin tin
- 8-inch baking dish
- 9-inch cake pan
- 9-inch pie plate
- 9-inch springform pan
- 11 × 7-inch baking dish
- 9 × 13-inch baking dish
- 10-inch cast-iron skillet
- 12-inch cast-iron skillet
- 10-inch nonstick sauté pan
- 12-inch nonstick sauté pan
- 10-inch stainless sauté pan
- 12-inch stainless sauté pan
- Large heavy-bottomed pot or Dutch oven
- Small saucepan
- Medium saucepan
- Small, medium, and large bowls
- Colander
- Mesh strainer
- Whisk
- Cookie scoop
- Ladle
- Vegetable peeler
- Citrus press
- Rubber spatula
- Wooden spoon
- Potato masher
- Dry measuring cups
- Liquid measuring cups
- Measuring spoons
- Pastry brush
- Blender
- Food processor
- Waffle iron
- Spiralizer
- Popsicle molds
- Box grater
- Microplane
- Chef's knife
- Paring knife
- Cutting board
- Baking sheets
- Parchment paper

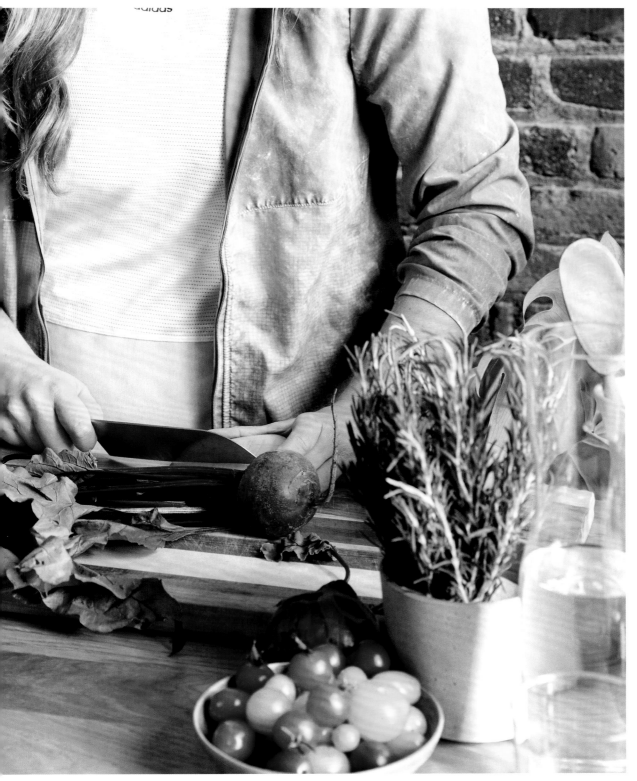

Meal Guides

Whenever I'm looking at a collection of recipes, I like to learn how to use the recipes to enhance both my health and fitness. In this chapter, you'll find two detailed meal plans to help identify how to use the recipes in this book, whether you're a high-performance or training athlete or someone who enjoys exercising a few times a week.

Because meal planning and shopping for recipes can often become overwhelming, I've also included a grocery list template of how I organize and shop to be sure I don't forget anything on a big haul from the store.

Meal Guide for the Endurance Athlete in Peak Training

This plan is designed for endurance athletes in peak training season, with a concentration on heavy training over the weekend. Post-workout snacks are essential to consume within 30 to 45 minutes after the workout since this is the critical window of repair and rebuilding for your body.

	Sunday	Monday	Tuesday	Wednesday	Thursday	Friday	Saturday
Workout	Long Ride (3+ hours)	Recovery Day Swim (easy swim, about 40 minutes)	Tempo Run (a fast-paced run for a longer period of time)	Easy Ride (about 1 hour 15 minutes)	Track Run (a shorter run with more intense intervals)	Rest Day	Long Run (1 hour 30 minutes)
Breakfast	Baked Pumpkin Quinoa with Apples and Figs (page 42)	Pre-swim: Date Bites (2 to 3 bites, page 191)	Leftover Baked Pumpkin Quinoa with Apples and Figs	Roasted "Smoked" Carrot Toast with Sesame-Crusted Egg and Dill (page 51)	Superfood Mixed-Berry Chia Jam (page 240) on toast + nut butter	Weekday Breakfast Burrito (page 44)	Almond Berry Overnight Oats (page 38)
Mid- or Post-workout Bite	Long-Ride Snack: Everything Bagel Trail Bar (page 201) + Date Bite (page 191)	Post-swim Meal: Gut-Healthy Brown Rice Bowl with Kimchi and Egg (page 41)	Post-run: Energized Mocha Crunch Smoothie (page 71)	Ride Snack: Peanut Butter Compost Cookie (page 188)	Post-run: Energized Mocha Crunch Smoothie (page 71)		Post-long run: Anti-Inflammatory Beet Mango Smoothie (page 79)
Lunch	Vegan Chickpea Kale Caesar (page 90) + protein of choice	Leftover Southwestern Vegetable Slow Cooker Chili + avocado	Leftover Hasselback Sweet Potatoes + two fried eggs and greens	Falafel Slider Greek Salad Bowl (page 105)	Thai Crunch Salad (page 96) + protein of choice	Leftover Portuguese Spicy White Bean Stew with Tomatoes and Kale + side salad	Leftover BBQ Fajita Bowl
Snack	Coconut Matcha Fat Bites (page 184)	Lemon Blueberry Muffin (page 48)	Roasted Garlic Green Hummus (page 161) + Veggies	Farmers' Market Smoothie (page 74)	Leftover Lemon Blueberry Muffin	Spiced Nuts Trail Mix (page 198) + apple	Date Nut Zucchini Bread (age 55)
Dinner	Southwestern Vegetable Slow Cooker Chili (page 94) + avocado and side salad	Ginger-Pineapple Salmon Burger (page 122) + Hasselback Sweet Potatoes with Mustard Seed and Yogurt (page 162)	Quinoa Crust Pizza with Broccoli Rabe and Almond Ricotta (page 135) + Supergreen Pesto herby sauce (page 112; double batch!) + baked tofu	Leftover Supergreen Pasta herby sauce + plant-based pasta + protein of choice	Portuguese Spicy White Bean Stew with Tomatoes and Kale (page 111) + Lemon Anchovy Broccolini (page 156)	BBQ-Fajita Bowl (page 89)	Soba Noodle Bowl with Tahini and Tofu (page 98) + side salad
Dessert	Apple Walnut Crisp (page 222) + peppermint tea	Almost Raw Chocolate Candy Bar (page 227) + ginger tea	Leftover Apple Walnut Crisp + herbal tea	Flourless Fudgy Black Bean Brownie (page 208) + mint tea	Pecan Pie Date Bite (page 193) + ginger tea	Cinnamon Crumb Coffee Cake (page 213) + peppermint tea	Leftover Flourless Fudgy Black Bean Brownie + ginger tea

Meal Guide for the Everyday Health-Conscious Person

This meal plan is for the everyday health-conscious person who is not necessarily training or practicing high-intensity workouts but is looking to eat clean whole foods. Each day of the plan is designed to keep you full to maintain stable energy levels for high daily living performance. Once again everyone is different, and these are just suggestions of meals to help plan your week.

	Sunday	Monday	Tuesday	Wednesday	Thursday	Friday	Saturday
Breakfast	Peanut Butter and Banana Pancakes with Chocolate Chips (page 47) + fresh fruit	Apricot and Almond Granola with Quinoa (page 56) + vegan yogurt and berries	Chocolate Almond Smoothie Bowl (page 73)	Leftover Apricot and Almond Granola with Quinoa + nut milk and fruit	Anti-Inflammatory Turmeric Tofu Mediterranean Scramble (page 45)	Date Nut Zucchini Bread (page 55) + Pumpkin Pie Smoothie (page 70)	Shakshuka with Crispy Chickpeas and Avocado (page 52)
Lunch	Broccoli Quinoa Salad with Apples and Almonds (page 104) + protein of choice	Leftover Vegan Asian Meat Loaf with Lentils and Shiitakes over greens	Supergreen Pasta (page 112)	Forbidden Rice Salad with Roasted Beets and Butternut Squash (page 114) + 2 hard-boiled eggs	Leftover Homemade BBQ Salmon + Cauliflower Mujadara (page 160)	Falafel Slider Greek Salad Bowl (page 105)	Leftover Falafel Slider Greek Salad Bowl
Snack	Spiced Nuts Trail Mix (page 198) + cut-up veggies	Chia Almond Coconut Bar (page 187)	Cookie Dough Date Bite (page 192)	Leftover Chia Almond Coconut Bar	Roasted Garlic Green Hummus (page 161) + veggies	Fig and Oat Bar (page 182)	Leftover Date Nut Zucchini Bread
Dinner	Vegan Asian Meat Loaf with Lentils and Shiitakes (page 137) + Miso-Mashed Sweet Potatoes with Ginger Shiitakes (page 153) + side salad	Pomegranate Pecan-Crusted Halibut with Brussels Sprouts and Lentils (page 132) + Braised Apple Dijon Cabbage (page 159)	Tempeh and Brussels Sprouts Tacos with Pickled Cabbage (page 124) + Vegan Mexican Street Corn (page 150) + side salad	Homemade BBQ Salmon (page 125) + Braised Swiss Chard and Kabocha Squash (page 167)	Sheet Pan Cauliflower and Sweet Potato Curry (page 136)	Spicy Peanut Tofu Pad Thai (page 93) + Chili-Spiced Crispy Brussels Sprouts (page 157)	Pasta with Vodka Cream Sauce (page 102) + Vegan Chickpea Kale Caesar (page 90)
Dessert	Nutty Tahini Fudge (page 210) + mint tea	Watermelon-Kiwi Ice Pops (page 218) + mint tea	Chocolate Chip Oat Cookie (page 217) + herbal tea	Carrot Cake with Cashew Cream Cheese Frosting (page 214) + ginger tea	Leftover Nutty Tahini Fudge + herbal tea	Lemon Raspberry Tart (page 221) + peppermint tea	Flourless Fudgy Black Bean Brownie (page 208) + ginger tea

Grocery List

canned foods
_____
_____
_____
_____
_____

carbohydrates
_____
_____
_____
_____
_____

baking needs
_____
_____
_____
_____

dairy
_____
_____
_____
_____
_____

snack foods
_____
_____
_____
_____
_____

protein sources
_____
_____
_____
_____

frozen foods
_____
_____
_____
_____
_____

produce
_____
_____
_____
_____

condiments
_____
_____
_____
_____

breakfast/cereals
_____
_____
_____
_____

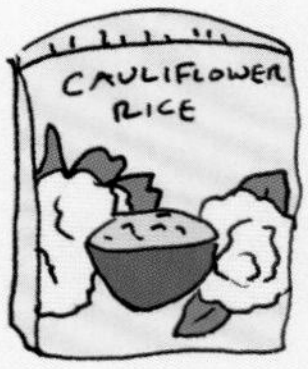

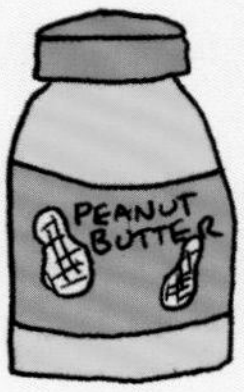

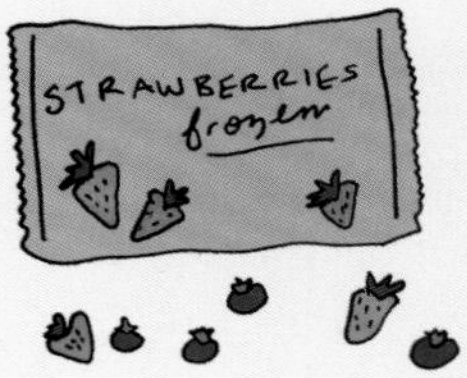

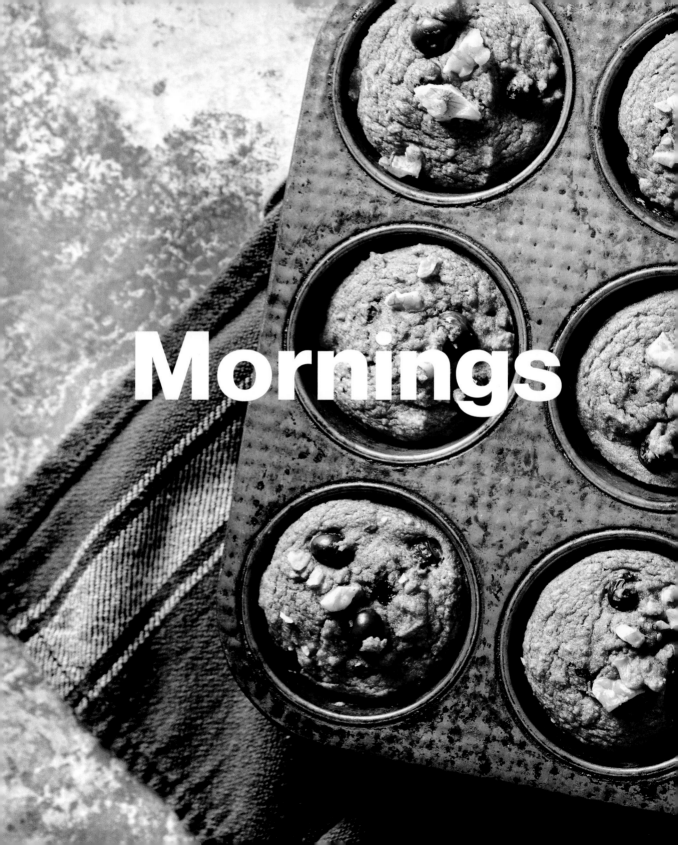

Mornings

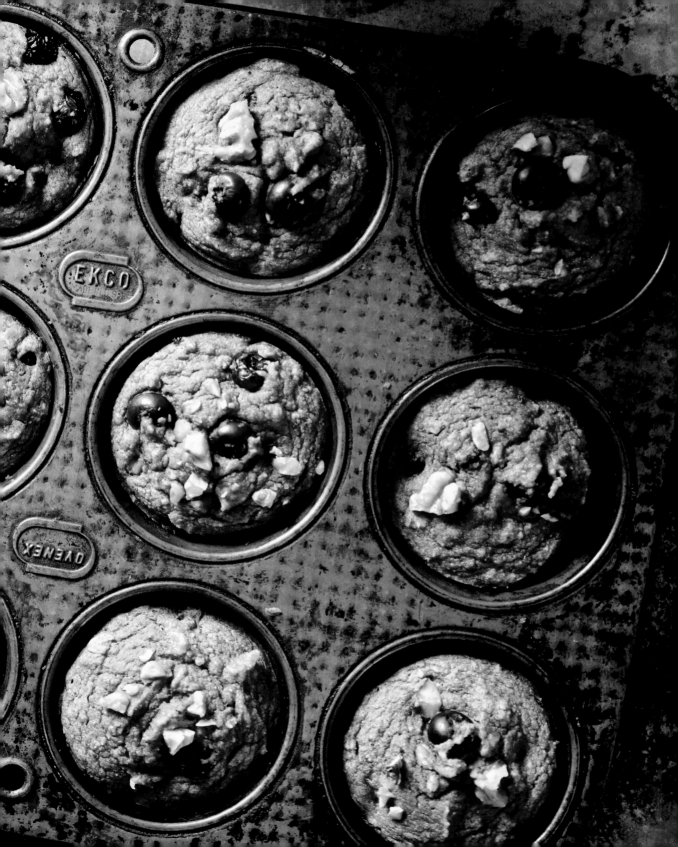

Starting my day off right is always what keeps me on track and fueled for the day. If you eat a filling breakfast full of vitamins and nutrients, you'll have the energy you need to get off to a nourishing start and get through the morning. Breakfast is something I always get excited about, so I've shared my top-choice recipes here to help inspire you. Some of my favorites are the Almond Berry Overnight Oats (page 38) as a meal-prep trick, Weekday Breakfast Burrito (page 44) for mornings I'm working from home, and Shakshuka with Crispy Chickpeas and Avocado (page 52) for a Sunday brunch with friends.

One question athletes and friends regularly ask me about making breakfast is, "If I want something sweeter in the mornings, how can I do this in a healthier way that won't make me hungry or cause my blood sugar to spike?" My philosophy is to always use natural sweeteners and avoid any added sweeteners. I sweeten naturally using dates and fresh fruit for breakfast time—fruit already has so much flavor and delicious sweetness to add to any recipe, and it will keep you feeling great whether you are heading to work or school or eating before or after a workout. Try the Baked Pumpkin Quinoa with Apples and Figs (page 42) or the Lemon Blueberry Muffins (page 48) and you'll see what I mean!

Almond Berry Overnight Oats

PREP TIME// 5 minutes

COOK TIME// 2 minutes + refrigeration overnight

SERVES// 1

1 cup unsweetened nut milk

2 tablespoons Superfood Mixed-Berry Chia Jam (page 240)

½ cup old-fashioned rolled oats

1 teaspoon chia seeds

¼ teaspoon ground cinnamon

¼ teaspoon vanilla extract

Pinch of sea salt

1 tablespoon unsweetened natural almond butter, to garnish

Raspberries and blueberries, to garnish

Chopped toasted almonds, to garnish

When I know I'm going to have a crazy week, and breakfast becomes an afterthought, I make these overnight oats ahead of time. This is an easy pantry-staple recipe perfect to eat before heading out for a workout. Use your favorite fruit as well as naturally sweetened jam, like my Superfood Mixed Berry Chia Jam (page 240), to make endless combinations.

1 In a small saucepan, heat the nut milk until simmering. Meanwhile, place the jam in a pint-size mason jar. Top with the oats, chia seeds, cinnamon, vanilla, and salt. Pour the warm nut milk over the top and stir to combine. Cover with a lid and place in the refrigerator overnight.

2 Before serving, stir the oat mixture again, then top with almond butter, fresh berries, and toasted almonds.

TIP: Oats are a great complex carbohydrate to eat before a morning workout. Soaking the oats overnight helps break down their natural enzymes, making them easier to digest. For this recipe, I heat the milk before pouring it over the oats for maximum absorption, making the oats thick and creamy in the morning.

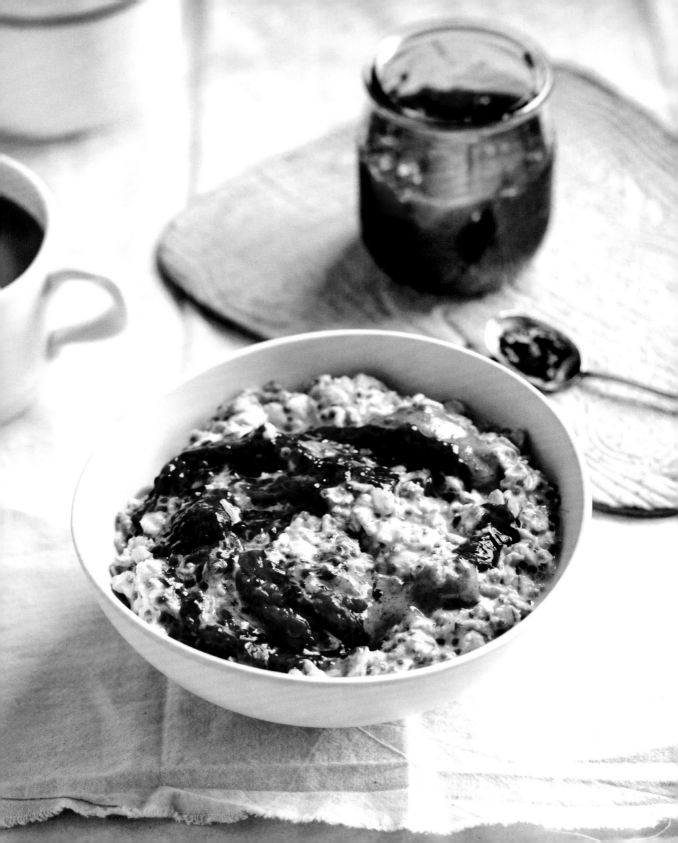

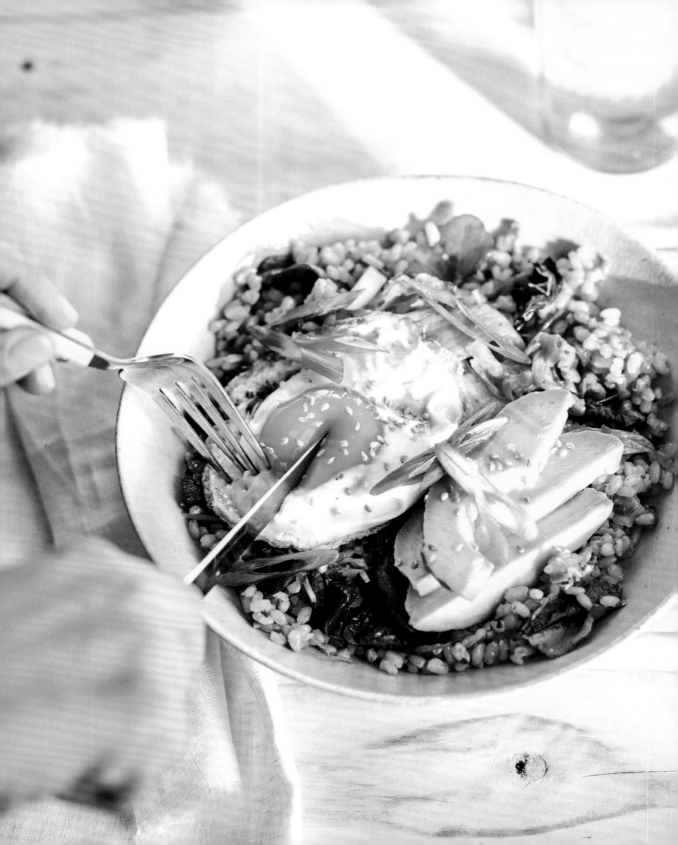

Gut-Healthy Brown Rice Bowl

with Kimchi and Egg

PREP TIME// 10 minutes

COOK TIME// 45 minutes

SERVES// 1

Rice Base

1 tablespoon toasted sesame oil

2 scallions (white and light green parts), minced

1 garlic clove, minced

1 (1-inch) piece ginger, peeled and grated

½ cup brown rice

½ teaspoon sea salt

1 cup water

1 cup baby kale

Bowl Toppings

1 tablespoon avocado oil

1 large egg

2 tablespoons chopped store-bought kimchi

2 teaspoons toasted sesame seeds

1 scallion (white and light green parts), thinly sliced

¼ avocado, pitted, peeled, and thinly sliced

Pinch of sea salt

Sometimes a savory breakfast is exactly what I'm craving. This bowl is full of gut-healthy benefits from the kimchi. Kimchi comes from Korea and is fermented cabbage with several other seasonings. It was originally used as a food preservation method but now is known for its unique sour and often spicy flavor as well as health benefits. It's made by lacto-fermentation, which starts with a salt brine to kill bad bacteria, then uses the remaining good bacteria to convert sugars into lactic acid. Kimchi contains probiotics, which help improve gut health as well as boost the immune system, making it a great way to start your day.

1 **For the Rice Base:** In a medium saucepan, heat the sesame oil over medium-high heat. Add the scallions, garlic, and ginger and allow to cook for 2 minutes, until fragrant. Add the rice and allow to toast for an additional minute. Season with salt. Add water, bring to a boil, then reduce the heat and allow to simmer, partially covered, according to rice package instructions.

2 Once the rice is cooked, fluff with a fork and stir in the kale, allowing the heat from the rice to lightly wilt the greens. Set aside.

3 **For the Bowl Toppings:** In a small nonstick sauté pan, heat the avocado oil over medium heat. Crack the egg into a small bowl and then carefully slide the egg into the pan. Allow to cook for 3 to 4 minutes, until the white is set but the yolk is still runny. Remove from the heat.

4 Place the rice base in a bowl and top with the kimchi, sesame seeds, scallion, avocado, salt, and the fried egg. Serve.

TIP: If you ever have leftover brown rice, feel free to use it in this recipe. Just sauté the cooked rice with the scallions, garlic, and ginger until warmed through and aromatic.

Baked Pumpkin Quinoa

with Apples and Figs

PREP TIME// 10 minutes

COOK TIME// 50 minutes

SERVES// 4 to 6

2 teaspoons coconut oil, for greasing

2 small tart red apples, such as Honeycrisp, peeled and diced small

1 lemon, juiced

1 (15-ounce) can unsweetened pumpkin puree

2 large eggs, beaten

2 cups unsweetened nut milk

1 teaspoon ground cinnamon

¼ teaspoon ground nutmeg

¼ teaspoon ground cloves

Pinch of sea salt

1 cup quinoa, rinsed

⅓ cup dried Turkish figs, chopped, plus additional chopped to garnish

½ cup toasted pecans, chopped, to garnish

This is my ultimate breakfast recipe for the fall, and it's perfect for sharing as a brunch or making as a meal-prep breakfast for the whole week. The pumpkin puree adds a natural sweetness and creamy texture to the protein-packed nutty quinoa. This elevated morning bake also makes your home smell amazing!

1 Preheat the oven to 350°F. Lightly grease a 9 × 9-inch baking dish with the coconut oil.

2 In a small bowl, toss the apples in the lemon juice and set aside. In a large bowl, whisk together the pumpkin puree, eggs, nut milk, cinnamon, nutmeg, cloves, and salt. Fold the apples into the mixture.

3 Place the rinsed quinoa in the bottom of the prepared baking dish and sprinkle with the chopped figs. Top with the pumpkin puree mixture. Bake for 45 to 50 minutes, or until the top is set. Remove from the oven and allow to cool for 10 minutes. Garnish with additional chopped figs and toasted pecans.

SERVING TIP: I sometimes like to serve this quinoa with warm nut milk on the side to pour over once served in bowls.

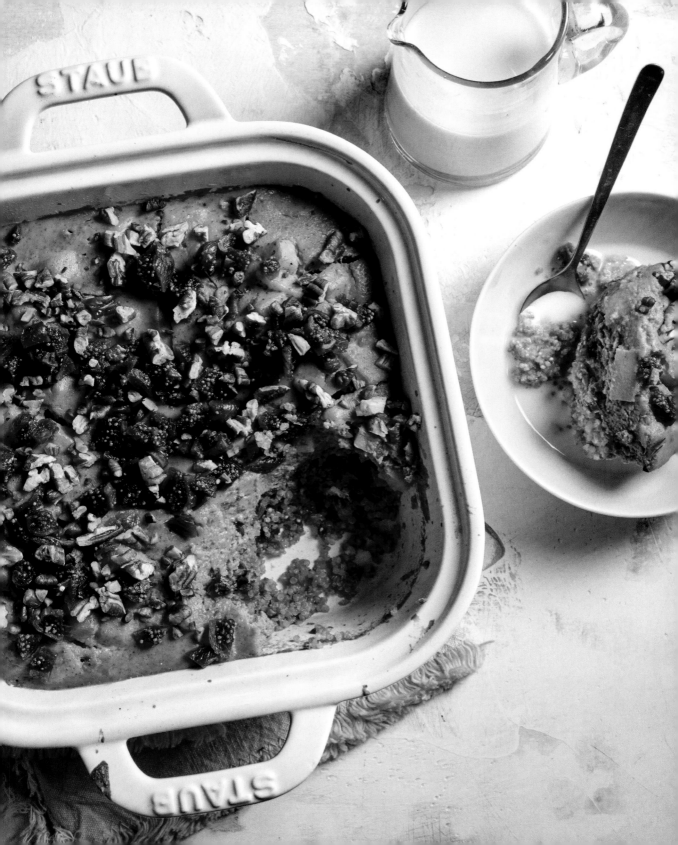

Weekday
Breakfast Burrito

PREP TIME// 10 minutes

COOK TIME// 15 minutes

SERVES// 4

2 tablespoons avocado oil

1 red bell pepper, cored, seeded, and diced

1 medium red onion, diced small

1 (15-ounce) can black beans, drained and rinsed

Pinch of cayenne pepper

Sea salt and freshly ground black pepper to taste

4 large eggs plus 4 large egg whites, or 1 (12-ounce) package regular tofu, drained and pressed (see step 1, page 45)

4 cups packed baby spinach

4 brown rice burrito tortillas, warmed, or 8 large collard green leaves, stems removed

½ cup store-bought fresh salsa

Hot sauce of choice (optional)

1 avocado, pitted, peeled, and thinly sliced

This burrito is inspired by one that I get at my local bodega in New York City and is easy enough to make on a weekday morning. I like to customize my burrito with my favorite veggies and protein depending on what I'm craving. Feel free to use eggs or tofu as the protein; for the wrapper, I like to use either a brown rice tortilla or collard green leaf.

1   In a large nonstick sauté pan, heat the avocado oil over medium-high heat. Add the bell pepper and onion and allow to cook for 6 to 7 minutes, until softened and lightly browned. Add the black beans and cayenne and season with salt and pepper.

2   In a medium bowl, whisk together the eggs and egg whites and season with salt and pepper. Add the eggs to the pan and reduce the heat to medium. Slowly stir with a rubber spatula until small curds begin to form. Once the eggs are about halfway cooked through, 3 minutes or so, add the spinach in batches and stir, allowing the leaves to wilt from the heat. Season once more with salt and pepper.

3   Place a burrito tortilla on the counter in front of you and spread the tortilla with some of the salsa. Top with some of the eggs, hot sauce, if desired, and a couple of slices of avocado. Fold the two short sides of the burrito tortilla inward, then fold the side closest to you over the filling and continue rolling until a burrito is formed. Repeat with remaining tortillas and filling. Slice burritos in half and serve.

For the Collard Green Wrap:

Follow steps 1 and 2 above, then prepare an ice water bath. Bring a large pot of salted water to a boil. Add the collard green leaves a couple at a time and allow to wilt for 20 to 30 seconds, or until tender. Immediately remove the leaves from the boiling water and place in the ice water bath to cool. Remove from the cold water and pat dry. Repeat with remaining collard green leaves.

Make a burrito shell by overlapping the stemmed part of two collard green leaves to become a large burrito wrapper. Assemble burrito as described in step 3 above and serve.

Anti-Inflammatory Turmeric Tofu Mediterranean Scramble

PREP TIME // 15 minutes +
10 minutes draining
COOK TIME // 17 minutes
SERVES // 4

Tofu Scramble

1 (12-ounce) package firm tofu, drained

2 tablespoons avocado oil

1 medium red onion, diced small

2 garlic cloves, minced

½ teaspoon ground turmeric

¼ teaspoon ground coriander

¼ teaspoon dried oregano

Sea salt and freshly ground black pepper to taste

2 cups cherry tomatoes, halved

2 cups packed baby spinach

2 whole wheat pitas, warmed and cut in half

¼ cup pitted Kalamata olives, chopped

2 tablespoons chopped fresh flat-leaf parsley

2 tablespoons chopped fresh dill

Tahini Sauce

¼ cup tahini, well stirred

3 tablespoons fresh lemon juice

¼ cup water

This scramble looks just like eggs, thanks to its natural yellow color from the turmeric. In order for the body to benefit from all the powerful anti-inflammatory properties of turmeric, there needs to be black pepper. Black pepper has a compound called piperine that stops the breakdown of turmeric by the liver and gut, letting higher levels of turmeric remain in the body. I love making this simple Mediterranean scramble as a luxurious weekend breakfast, but I can also pack it into a pita pocket for an easy portable weekday meal.

1 **For the Tofu Scramble:** Line a plate with paper towels. Place the tofu on top of the paper towels and place more paper towels on top of the tofu. Place a heavy pan on top of the tofu and allow the tofu to drain of excess liquid for 10 minutes. Pat very dry.

2 In a large nonstick sauté pan, heat the avocado oil over medium heat. Add the onion and garlic and cook for about 4 minutes, or until softened. Add the turmeric, coriander, and oregano and cook for an additional minute. Season with salt and pepper. Add the tomatoes and cook for another 2 minutes. Crumble the tofu into the pan and allow to cook through for 7 to 10 minutes. Add the spinach during the last 3 minutes of cooking and stir until wilted. Season with salt and pepper.

3 **For the Tahini Sauce:** In a small bowl, whisk together the tahini, lemon juice, and water until smooth. Set aside.

4 Open a pita and stuff with tofu scramble. Sprinkle with olives, parsley, dill, and a drizzle of the tahini sauce. Repeat with the remaining pita halves.

TIP: Feel free to use eggs for this recipe as well: 6 large eggs plus 2 egg whites is perfect. Stir the eggs constantly until small curds form.

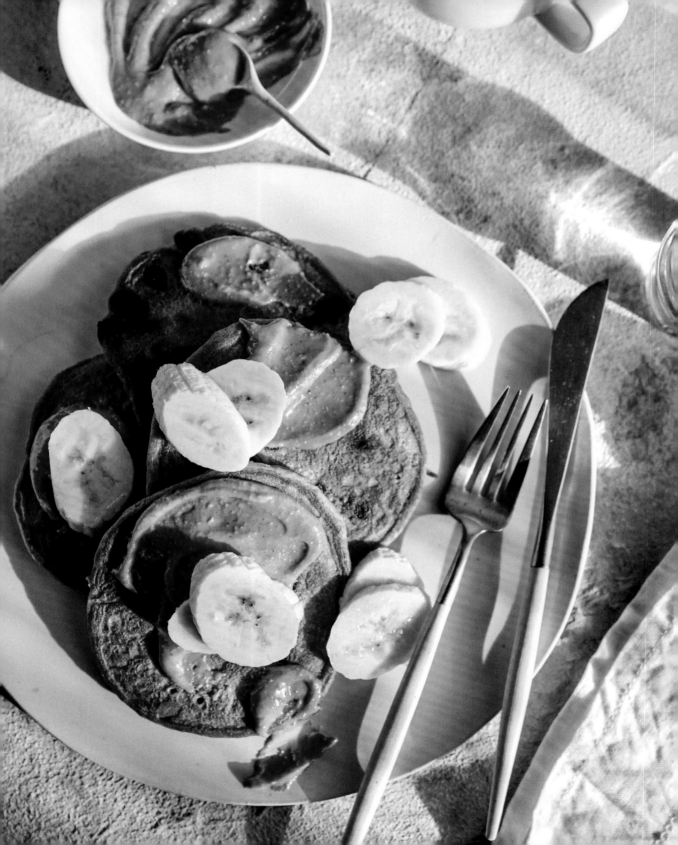

Peanut Butter
and Banana Pancakes

with Chocolate Chips

PREP TIME// 15 minutes

COOK TIME// 20 minutes

SERVES// 4

2 cups oat flour

½ cup almond flour

2 teaspoons ground cinnamon

2 teaspoons baking powder

½ teaspoon baking soda

½ teaspoon sea salt

2 bananas, peeled and mashed
(about ¾ cup)

⅓ cup unsweetened natural creamy
peanut butter

2 large eggs, lightly beaten

2 teaspoons vanilla extract

2 cups unsweetened nut milk

½ cup stevia-sweetened dark
chocolate chips (I like Lily's)

Coconut oil cooking spray, for
greasing

Optional Toppings

1 to 2 bananas, peeled and thinly sliced

Unsweetened natural creamy peanut
butter

Unsweetened applesauce

These are my go-to pancakes. They are not only easy to make, but they also taste delicious. They're naturally sweetened with the bananas, so there's no added sugar, making them a favorite in the morning, and the peanut butter provides protein. Almond and oat flour not only keep the pancakes gluten-free but also make the consistency light and fluffy from their fine textures. In the summer, I like to use berries rather than chocolate chips for a seasonal twist!

1   In a large bowl, whisk together the oat flour, almond flour, cinnamon, baking powder, baking soda, and salt.

2   In a medium bowl, whisk together the mashed bananas, peanut butter, eggs, and vanilla until smooth. Add the nut milk and whisk again until incorporated. Make a well in the flour mixture and pour the banana mixture into the well, stirring to combine. Fold in the chocolate chips.

3   Grease a large nonstick sauté pan with cooking spray and place over medium-low heat. Add ¼ cup of the pancake batter to the pan and allow to cook for 2 to 3 minutes, until golden brown and small bubbles begin forming on the top. Flip and cook for another 2 to 3 minutes, until golden brown on the second side and cooked through. Repeat with remaining pancake batter to make 16 pancakes total.

4   Feel free to top your pancakes with sliced banana, more peanut butter, or unsweetened applesauce.

TIPS: If you want to turn this recipe into waffles, use ½ cup unsweetened nut milk in total.

Try adding protein powder to these pancakes. Add 2 tablespoons unflavored, vanilla, or chocolate protein powder and whisk until smooth.

Lemon Blueberry Muffins

PREP TIME// 15 minutes +
15 minutes soaking
COOK TIME// 20 minutes
MAKES// 12 muffins

Coconut oil cooking spray, for greasing

1 cup pitted Medjool dates, halved

Hot water (115°F to 120°F), to cover dates

1¼ cups oat flour

¾ cup almond flour

½ cup old-fashioned rolled oats

1 tablespoon ground flaxseed

½ teaspoon sea salt

2 teaspoons ground cinnamon

1 teaspoon baking soda

½ cup unsweetened nut milk

½ cup unsweetened applesauce

1 teaspoon vanilla extract

1 tablespoon coconut oil, melted

1 lemon, zested

3 tablespoons fresh lemon juice

2 large eggs, lightly beaten

1 cup blueberries, saving a few for topping

¼ cup walnuts, chopped, saving a few for topping

This muffin is the perfect pre-workout breakfast with its not-too-sweet bran flavor. I like making a big batch of these muffins and storing them in the fridge for my busy mornings. In this version, I've flavored my muffins with lemon, blueberries, and walnuts, but feel free to customize the flavors with different nuts, fruit, or stevia-sweetened chocolate chips.

1 Preheat the oven to 350°F. Grease a 12-cup muffin tin with cooking spray.

2 In a small heatproof bowl, cover the dates with hot water and allow to soak for 15 minutes to soften. Drain and discard the liquid.

3 In a large bowl, whisk together the oat flour, almond flour, oats, flaxseed, salt, cinnamon, and baking soda.

4 Transfer the softened dates to the bowl of a food processor fitted with the blade attachment and add the nut milk, applesauce, vanilla, melted coconut oil, lemon zest, and lemon juice. Blend until smooth. Add the eggs and pulse until just combined.

5 Add half the flour mixture to the food processor and pulse until just incorporated. Add the remaining half of the flour mixture and pulse again (be careful not to overmix!). Scrape the batter into a bowl and fold in the blueberries and walnuts.

6 Fill each greased muffin cup two-thirds full. Sprinkle the tops with some of the reserved blueberries and walnuts. Bake for 18 to 20 minutes, or until golden brown and an inserted toothpick comes out clean. Allow to cool in the pan for 10 minutes, then remove and allow to cool completely. Store in an airtight container in the refrigerator for up to 3 days.

TIP: Try toasting the muffins and topping with your favorite unsweetened nut butter.

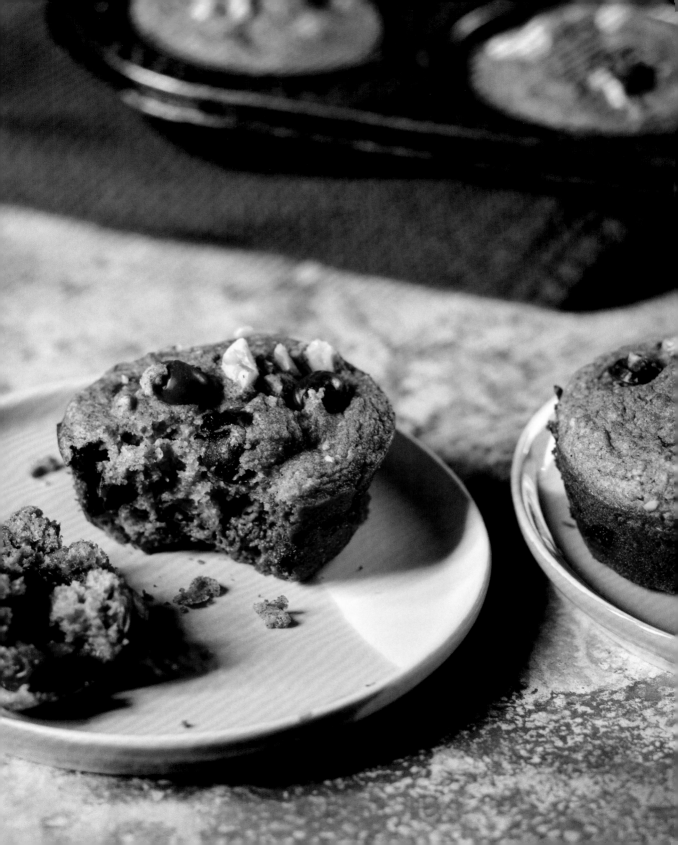

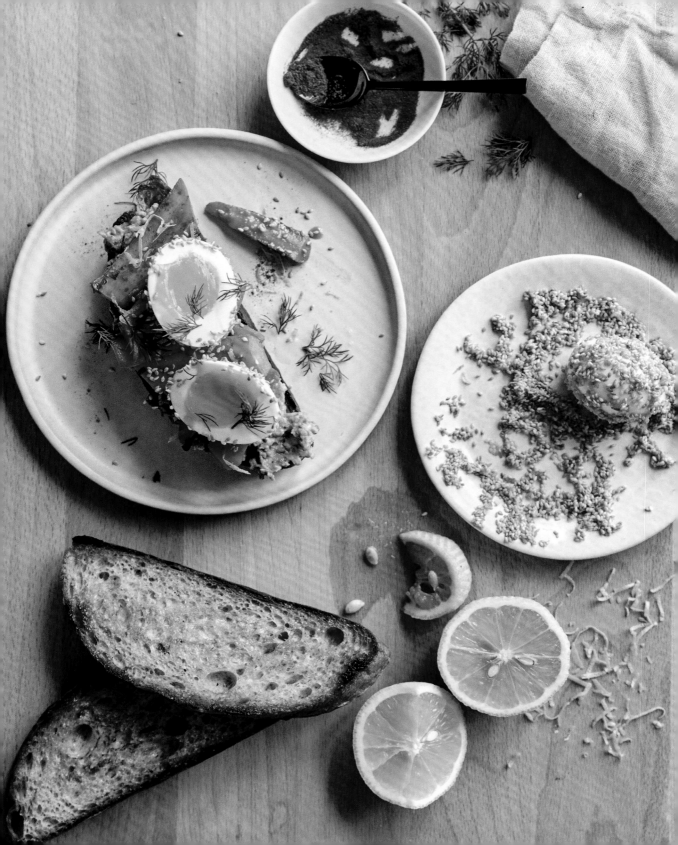

Roasted "Smoked" Carrot Toast

with Sesame-Crusted Egg and Dill

PREP TIME// 10 minutes +
marinating for at least 1 hour or
up to overnight

COOK TIME// 45 minutes

SERVES// 2

"Smoked" Carrot Toast

3 or 4 rainbow or regular carrots

2 tablespoons avocado oil

Salt to taste

1 tablespoon caper brine (you can also use olive or pickle brine)

¼ cup rice wine vinegar

1 tablespoon white miso paste

1 tablespoon liquid aminos (I like Bragg)

¼ teaspoon smoked paprika, plus additional to garnish

1 avocado, pitted and peeled

3 tablespoons fresh lemon juice

2 slices whole wheat sourdough bread

Lemon zest, to garnish

Fresh dill, to garnish

Sesame-Crusted Egg

2 large eggs

2 tablespoons toasted sesame seeds

This toast is inspired by something similar that I ate on a trip to Iceland a few years ago. Marinating tender carrots in the caper brine mixture brings out a salty, smoky flavor almost like lox. I always like to top toast with a runny boiled egg, and this one I happen to coat in sesame seeds for a crunchy, nutty flavor on the outside.

1 **For the "Smoked" Carrot Toast:** Preheat the oven to 400°F. Line a baking sheet with parchment paper.

2 Toss carrots with avocado oil. Season with salt. Place on the prepared baking sheet and roast for 40 to 45 minutes, until tender, flipping halfway through. Allow to cool completely.

3 Meanwhile, in a medium bowl, whisk together the caper brine, vinegar, miso paste, liquid aminos, and paprika. Once the carrots have cooled, cut into several ¼-inch strips that are about 3 inches long (like sushi sashimi). Add the carrots to the caper brine mixture and allow to marinate for at least 1 hour and up to overnight.

4 **For the Sesame-Crusted Egg:** Bring a small saucepan of water to a boil over medium-high heat. Prepare an ice water bath. Add the eggs gently into the water and boil for 7 minutes. Immediately place the eggs into the ice water bath and allow to cool completely. Carefully peel the eggs.

5 Place the sesame seeds on a plate. Roll the outside of the eggs in the sesame seeds. Set aside until ready to serve.

6 When ready to serve, in a small bowl, mash the avocado with 2 tablespoons of the lemon juice. Season with salt. Toast the bread. Gently spread the avocado mash on both pieces of toast. Top with the marinated carrots and garnish with the lemon zest, the remaining 1 tablespoon lemon juice, fresh dill, and a sprinkle of smoked paprika. Slice the eggs in half and place on top right before serving.

Shakshuka

with Crispy Chickpeas and Avocado

PREP TIME// 10 minutes

COOK TIME// 38 minutes

SERVES// 4

2 tablespoons avocado oil

1 medium red onion, diced

2 garlic cloves, minced

1 (15-ounce) can chickpeas, drained, rinsed, and patted dry

1 red bell pepper, cored, seeded, and chopped

Sea salt and freshly ground black pepper to taste

2 teaspoons cumin seed

1 teaspoon ground coriander

1 teaspoon sweet paprika

Pinch of cayenne pepper (optional)

1 tablespoon tomato paste

1 (28-ounce) can crushed tomatoes

4 large eggs

¼ cup pitted Kalamata olives, chopped

2 tablespoons chopped fresh flat-leaf parsley

2 tablespoons chopped fresh dill

1 avocado, pitted, peeled, and thinly sliced

4 slices whole wheat sourdough bread, toasted, to serve

Shakshuka is a recipe that has been very popular the past few years. It's no wonder because it's healthy, flavorful, and easy to make. My version has an ingredient twist of chickpeas for added texture and protein. I like to make this recipe when I host a post-workout group brunch. I make the sauce ahead of time and then reheat it and freshly cook the eggs when guests arrive.

1 In a large cast-iron skillet or heavy-bottomed pan, heat the avocado oil over medium-high heat. Add the onion and garlic and cook for about 4 minutes, or until softened. Add the chickpeas and bell pepper and allow to cook for about 10 minutes, until the chickpeas begin to pop and become slightly crispy. Season with salt and pepper.

2 Add the cumin seed, coriander, paprika, cayenne, and tomato paste and cook another minute to caramelize. Add the tomatoes, then reduce the heat and allow to simmer for 10 minutes, or until the sauce has thickened slightly.

3 Make four wells in the tomato mixture. Crack one of the eggs into a small bowl and then carefully slide the egg into one of the wells. Repeat with the remaining eggs. Cover the pan and allow to simmer for 10 to 12 minutes, until the whites are set but the yolks are still runny.

4 Sprinkle with the chopped olives, parsley, and dill. Shingle the avocado slices over the top. Serve with sourdough toast.

TIP: To bring out the rich flavor of the tomato paste, it's best to always cook it for a minute or so with the spices to allow the natural sugars of the tomato to caramelize and add a rich, slightly sweet tomato flavor to any dish.

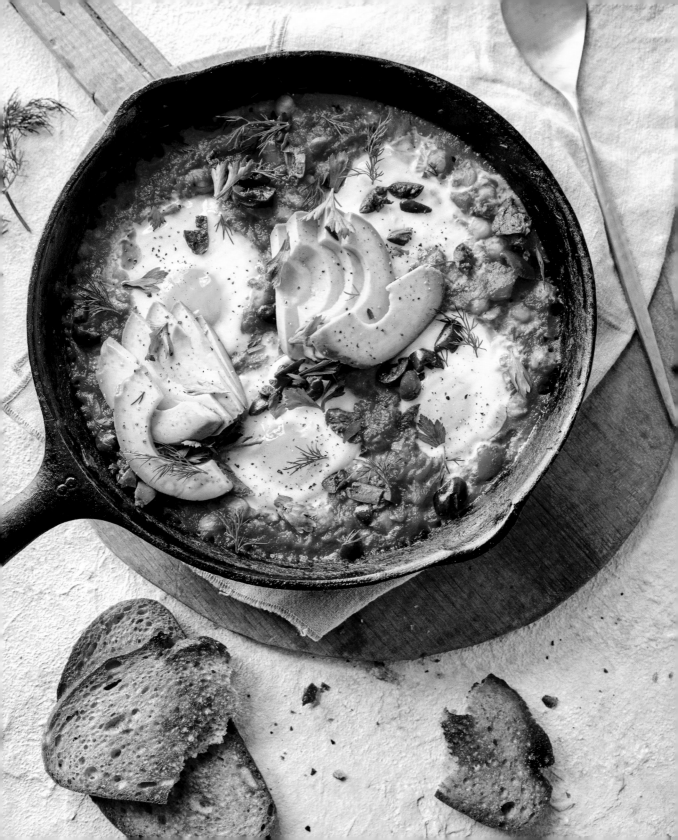

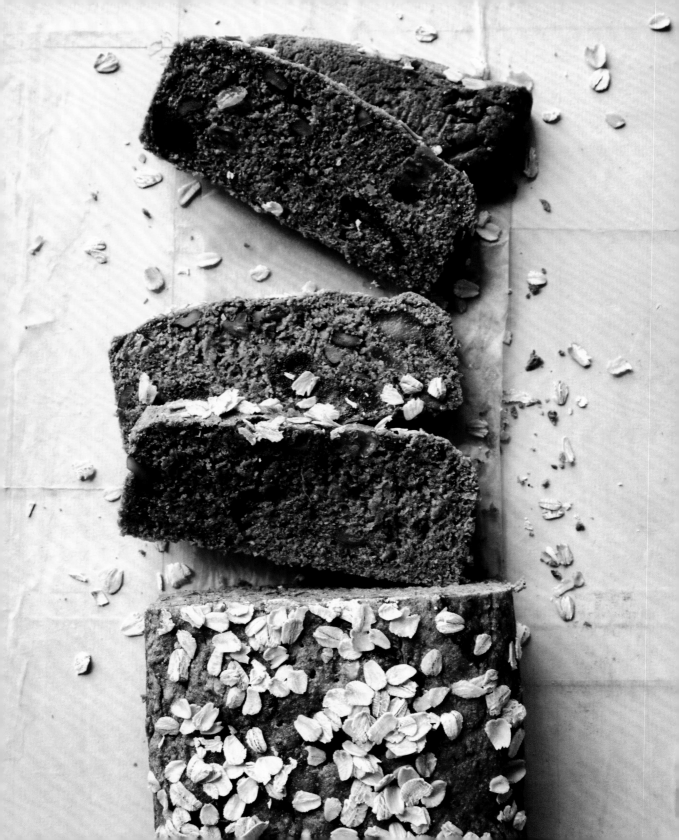

Date Nut Zucchini Bread

PREP TIME // 20 minutes +
15 minutes soaking

COOK TIME // 50 minutes

MAKES // one 9 × 5-inch loaf

¼ cup coconut oil, melted, plus additional for greasing

1 cup pitted Medjool dates, halved, plus ¼ cup, finely chopped

Hot water (115°F to 120°F), to cover dates

1½ cups white whole wheat flour

1½ teaspoons ground cinnamon

½ teaspoon ground nutmeg

¼ teaspoon ground cloves

1 teaspoon baking powder

½ teaspoon baking soda

½ teaspoon sea salt

½ cup unsweetened nut milk

2 teaspoons vanilla extract

1 tablespoon chia seeds

1 cup grated zucchini

½ cup walnuts, chopped

¼ cup golden raisins

2 tablespoons old-fashioned rolled oats

This dense zucchini nut bread is not only naturally sweetened, it's also vegan. I'm a big advocate of using whole fruits, like dates, to sweeten breakfast foods and add some fiber to start the day. I love bringing this bread to a brunch or group event because it's always a crowd-pleaser. The zucchini and dates keep the bread moist and lightly sweetened, while the warm spices are exactly what I'm craving in the morning with my coffee. Plus, the oats, chopped dates, walnuts, and raisins are some of my key textural flavors to add to a nut bread.

1 Preheat the oven to 325°F. Lightly grease a 9 × 5-inch loaf pan with coconut oil and line with parchment paper. Allow the parchment paper to hang over the sides for easy removal.

2 In a small heatproof bowl, cover the halved dates with hot water and allow to soak for 15 minutes to soften. Drain and discard the liquid.

3 In a large bowl, whisk together the flour, cinnamon, nutmeg, cloves, baking powder, baking soda, and salt.

4 Transfer the softened dates to the bowl of a food processor fitted with the blade attachment and add the nut milk, coconut oil, vanilla, and chia seeds. Blend until smooth, scraping down the sides of the bowl as needed.

5 Make a well in the flour mixture and pour the date puree into the well. Add the grated zucchini to the flour mixture and stir everything until just combined (you may need to use your hands to mix because the dough will be thick). Add the chopped dates, walnuts, and raisins and fold gently to combine. Scrape the batter into the loaf pan. Sprinkle with the oats.

6 Cover with foil and bake for 20 minutes. Remove the foil and bake for another 30 minutes, or until an inserted toothpick comes out clean. Allow to cool for 20 minutes in the pan, then remove to a baking rack to cool completely. Place in an airtight container in the refrigerator for up to 3 days.

TIPS: This bread is also sturdy enough to bring on an outing or workout as an adventure snack. I often pack mine for a winter workout when I'm craving baked goods with warm spices.

For serving, try toasting this zucchini bread and topping with almond butter for added protein and a breakfast that is so delicious.

Apricot and Almond Granola

with Quinoa

PREP TIME// 15 minutes +
15 minutes soaking

COOK TIME// 35 minutes

MAKES// 5½ cups (8 servings)

1½ cups pitted Medjool dates, halved

Hot water (115°F to 120°F), to cover dates

2 cups old-fashioned rolled oats

1 cup quinoa

1 cup raw almonds, roughly chopped

½ cup ground flaxseed

½ cup raw pumpkin seeds

⅓ cup unsweetened natural almond butter

1 tablespoon vanilla extract

¼ cup coconut oil, melted

2 teaspoons ground cinnamon

1 teaspoon ground nutmeg

1 teaspoon sea salt

½ cup dried apricots, chopped

A good granola recipe is always important to have in your cooking repertoire. This granola is different because I use a date puree to naturally sweeten the ingredients rather than sugar. By coating the oats and nuts with a date puree and almond butter mixture, it forms clusters after baking. I add savory quinoa for a whole grain protein boost as well as pumpkin seeds for crunch and healthy fats.

1 Preheat the oven to 325°F. Line two baking sheets with parchment paper.

2 In a small heatproof bowl, cover the dates with hot water and allow to soak for 15 minutes to soften. Reserve the liquid.

3 Meanwhile, in a large bowl, combine the oats, quinoa, almonds, flaxseed, and pumpkin seeds.

4 Transfer the softened dates and their liquid to the bowl of a food processor fitted with the blade attachment and add the almond butter, vanilla, coconut oil, cinnamon, nutmeg, and salt. Pulse until smooth.

5 Pour over the oat mixture and toss to evenly coat. Spread between the two prepared baking sheets. Bake for 30 to 35 minutes, stirring halfway through, until golden and set.

6 Remove from the oven and add the apricots while granola is still warm, stirring with a spatula to combine. Allow to cool completely, then break into clusters. Store in an airtight container at room temperature for up to 1 week.

TIPS: Try eating this granola with unsweetened nut milk and berries in the morning before a workout.

I like using dates rather than maple syrup as a natural sweetener for breakfast recipes. Dates are a whole food and add more nutrients and fiber to start the day.

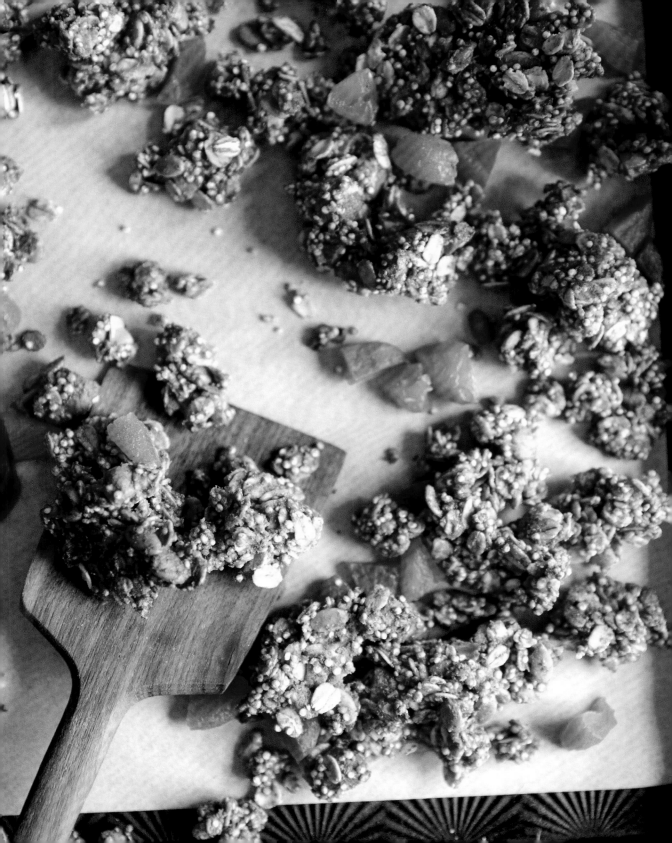

Summer Vegan Chickpea Frittata

PREP TIME// 10 minutes

COOK TIME// 1 hour 5 minutes

SERVES// 6

1½ cups chickpea flour

¼ cup nutritional yeast

1 teaspoon baking powder

1 teaspoon ground turmeric

1 teaspoon sea salt

1¾ cups water

¼ cup avocado oil

1 shallot, diced small

2 garlic cloves, minced

2 teaspoons chopped fresh thyme
or 1 teaspoon dried

1 teaspoon chopped fresh rosemary or
½ teaspoon dried

1 medium zucchini, cut into half-moons

1 cup cherry tomatoes, halved

Freshly ground black pepper to taste

1 cup packed baby arugula

This is the perfect summer brunch recipe for hosting a bunch of people. I love to head to the farmers' market early on weekend mornings to buy fresh seasonal vegetables to use in this frittata. In this version, I'm highlighting zucchini, tomatoes, and arugula. To make the recipe vegan, I use chickpea flour as the frittata base rather than egg. It's both creamy as well as slightly nutty in flavor, pairing nicely with sweet summer produce.

1 Preheat the oven to 375°F.

2 In a large bowl, whisk together the flour, nutritional yeast, baking powder, turmeric, and ½ teaspoon of the salt. Add water and whisk until smooth. Set aside.

3 In a 10-inch cast-iron skillet or nonstick sauté pan, heat 2 tablespoons of the avocado oil over medium heat. Add the shallot and garlic and cook for about 4 minutes, or until softened. Add the thyme, rosemary, zucchini, and tomatoes and cook for another 4 to 5 minutes, until the zucchini is lightly golden. Season with the remaining ½ teaspoon salt and the pepper, then add the arugula. Remove from the heat, tossing to allow the arugula to wilt, and allow to cool for 5 minutes.

4 Remove ½ cup of the cooked zucchini and tomatoes to a small bowl and set aside. Stir the remaining vegetable mixture into the chickpea batter. Grease the cast-iron skillet with the remaining 2 tablespoons avocado oil using a paper towel or heat-resistant brush. Pour the batter into the cast-iron skillet, sprinkle the top with the reserved ½ cup of cooked tomato and zucchini, and place in the oven. Bake for 35 to 40 minutes, until the top is set and an inserted toothpick in the center comes out clean. Remove from the oven and allow to cool for 10 minutes before serving.

TIP: If you prefer to use eggs, use 10 large eggs lightly beaten. Bake in the oven for 14 to 18 minutes, until the eggs are just set and the center slightly jiggles.

Tiffany Cromwell's Banana Bread

ATHLETE RECIPE: Tiffany Cromwell is an Australian professional cyclist with the Canyon/SRAM racing team on the Women's World Tour.

"I love having this banana bread as a training food to help fuel me, especially on long and hard training days. This banana bread is quite dense, and by adding oats and dates, it has plenty of clean energy that hits the spot when I'm in need of a boost. I also add walnuts or chocolate if I'm in the mood."

1 Preheat the oven to 350°F. Grease a 9 × 5-inch loaf pan with coconut oil.

2 In a small heatproof bowl, cover the dates with hot water and allow to soak for 15 minutes to soften. Drain and discard the liquid.

3 Transfer the softened dates to the bowl of a food processor fitted with the blade attachment and pulse until smooth. Add the coconut oil, egg, mashed banana, oat milk, and vanilla and blend until just combined and smooth.

4 In a large bowl, whisk together the flour, oats, baking soda, baking powder, cinnamon, and salt. Make a well in the center of the flour mixture and add the wet ingredient mixture. Mix until just combined. Add the walnuts or chocolate, if desired, and fold until just incorporated.

5 Scrape the batter into the loaf pan and smooth the top. Bake for 40 to 50 minutes, until golden brown and an inserted toothpick comes out clean. Cool in the pan on a wire baking rack. Slice and serve.

TIP: To make your own oat flour, in the bowl of a food processor fitted with the blade attachment, pulse 2 cups old-fashioned rolled oats until finely ground.

PREP TIME// 15 minutes + 1 hour soaking

COOK TIME// 50 minutes

SERVES// 8

¼ cup coconut oil, plus additional for greasing

1 cup pitted Medjool dates

Hot water (115°F to 120°F), to cover dates

1 large egg, lightly beaten

3 overripe bananas, mashed (about 1½ cups)

½ cup oat milk or other dairy-free milk alternative

1 teaspoon vanilla (from vanilla bean pod or vanilla extract)

1½ cups oat flour or alternative flour

1 cup old-fashioned rolled oats

2 teaspoons baking soda

1 teaspoon baking powder

2 teaspoons ground cinnamon

½ teaspoon sea salt

½ cup crushed walnuts or ½ cup high-quality dark chocolate, chopped (optional)

Colleen Quigley's Savory Sweet Potato Oat Bowl

with Tomatoes and Avocado

ATHLETE RECIPE: Colleen Quigley is an American distance runner specializing in the 3K steeplechase. She has represented Team USA in the 2015 and 2017 Outdoor World Championships, the 2018 Indoor World Championships (in the 1,500 meter), and the 2016 Olympic Games. Colleen graduated from Florida State University in 2015 with a bachelor's degree in dietetics and earned nine All-American honors during her time as a Seminole.

"For me, adding sweet potato to steel-cut oats for morning savory oats is a game changer! I used to be a fan of only sweet oats with berries, honey, and cinnamon, but then I began experimenting with savory oats for breakfast and haven't turned back! This oat bowl is perfect as my pre-workout breakfast. It keeps me fueled and doesn't upset my stomach during training. This is my favorite version of the recipe, but feel free to top yours with any of your favorite veggies."

1 For the Roasted Chickpeas: Preheat the oven to 425°F. Line a baking sheet with parchment paper.

2 Toss chickpeas with olive oil, salt, and pepper. Place on the prepared baking sheet and roast for 15 to 18 minutes, until crispy and lightly golden. Remove from the oven and allow to cool.

3 For the Oat Bowl: In a large pot or saucepan, bring to a boil the oats, sweet potato, and stock and season with salt. Reduce the heat and allow to simmer for 22 to 25 minutes, until the sweet potato is tender and the oats are cooked through.

4 Meanwhile, in a large nonstick sauté pan, heat the olive oil over medium heat. Crack one of the eggs into a small bowl and then carefully slide the egg into the pan. Repeat with the remaining eggs. Allow to cook for 4 to 5 minutes, until the whites solidify but the yolks are still runny.

5 Divide the oats among four bowls, top each with some tomatoes, avocado, chickpeas, an egg, and nutritional yeast. Season with additional salt and pepper, add toppings, if desired, and serve.

TIPS: Steel-cut are the least processed form of oats, which means they take the longest to cook. They have a chewy, nutty flavor. They are whole oats that have been chopped into pieces, which is where they get their texture. I like using steel-cut for oat bowls or savory recipes.

"I usually cook my oats and sweet potatoes ahead of time so that in the morning I only have to heat up the base and add the toppings. I also roast the chickpeas ahead of time and store them in an airtight container. If you want them extra-crunchy, pop them under the broiler for a minute or two in the morning before topping your oats."

—COLLEEN QUIGLEY

PREP TIME// 15 minutes
COOK TIME// 30 minutes
SERVES// 4

Roasted Chickpeas

1 (15-ounce) can chickpeas, drained, rinsed, and patted dry

1 tablespoon extra-virgin olive oil

¼ teaspoon sea salt

Freshly ground black pepper to taste

Oat Bowl

1 cup steel-cut oats

1 medium sweet potato, peeled and diced small (about 2 cups)

3 cups low-sodium vegetable stock

¼ teaspoon sea salt

1 tablespoon extra-virgin olive oil

4 large eggs

1 cup mixed cherry tomatoes, halved

1 avocado, pitted, peeled, and diced

2½ tablespoons nutritional yeast

Optional Toppings

Chopped roasted root vegetables, like beets or carrots

Wilted kale or spinach

Toasted nuts

Seeds

Emma Coburn's Apple Cinnamon French Toast

ATHLETE RECIPE: Emma Coburn is a professional track-and-field athlete and a three-time Olympian, World Champion, Olympic bronze medalist, eight-time US Champion, and World silver medalist in the 3,000-meter steeplechase. She was born and raised in Colorado and loves running on the beautiful roads and trails in her hometown, Crested Butte. In between her training runs, she loves to cook!

"I have quite the sweet tooth, and brunch is always my favorite meal, especially after a big run. With this recipe, I wanted to make a healthy French toast with an apple cinnamon sauce for topping. The apples give a great bite and good texture to the dish, and the cinnamon brings warmth that is extra appreciated after a cold run. This French toast is super simple and really delicious. Give it a try!"

1 For the Apple Cinnamon Sauce: In a small saucepan, heat the coconut oil over medium heat and add the apple. Cook for 3 to 5 minutes, until the apple starts to soften. Add the cinnamon, salt, and almond milk and stir. Reduce the heat to a simmer and cook for another 10 to 12 minutes, until the liquid starts to thicken. Remove from the heat, add the vanilla, and stir to combine. Cover to keep warm while making the French toast.

2 For the Almond Butter Drizzle: Melt the almond butter in the microwave for 45 seconds, stirring until loose and able to drizzle. Stir in the maple syrup. Set aside.

3 For the French Toast: In a shallow bowl, whisk together the egg, almond milk, cinnamon, nutmeg, and vanilla. Dip each bread slice in the egg mixture on each side until soaked through and place on a rack until ready to cook.

4 Grease a large nonstick sauté pan with cooking spray and place over medium heat. Add a couple of slices of the dipped bread. Reduce the heat to low and cover with a lid. Cook 2 minutes per side, or until golden brown. Repeat with the remaining slices of bread.

5 Place 2 slices of French toast on each plate and ladle the warm apple cinnamon sauce on top. Drizzle with the almond butter, if desired, and serve.

PREP TIME// 10 minutes
COOK TIME// 15 minutes
SERVES// 2

Apple Cinnamon Sauce

2 tablespoons coconut oil

1 medium sweet apple, such as Fuji or Gala, peeled, cored, and diced small

½ teaspoon ground cinnamon

¼ teaspoon sea salt

1 cup unsweetened almond milk

1 teaspoon vanilla extract

Optional Almond Butter Drizzle

1 to 2 tablespoons unsweetened natural almond butter

1 to 2 tablespoons pure maple syrup

French Toast

1 large egg

¼ cup unsweetened almond milk

½ teaspoon ground cinnamon

Pinch of nutmeg

1 teaspoon vanilla extract

4 slices sourdough bread

Coconut oil cooking spray, for greasing

Ayesha McGowan's Sweet Potato and Black Bean Sheet Pan Hash

ATHLETE RECIPE: Ayesha McGowan is a professional road cyclist for Liv Racing and an advocate for better representation of people of color in cycling. Upon entering competitive cycling in 2014, she quickly discovered that there had not been a single African American female pro road cyclist. She recently became the first. Through launching various initiatives that focus on diversity and representation in the sport of cycling, including her "Do Better Together" virtual ride series, Ayesha has inspired countless people, particularly people of color, to ride their bikes more often—both competitively and recreationally. Her work also encourages people of all backgrounds to challenge themselves and who they picture when they define the word *cyclist*.

"Figuring out what to eat was an extremely challenging part of my journey in cycling. There were times when I was so worried about what to eat that I lost my appetite altogether. Eventually, I discovered the best way for me to fuel for training and racing was to find ingredients that made me excited about eating. If a bite of something caused me to happy-dance, then it was perfect. Sweet potatoes always bring me joy and keep me dancing in the kitchen. I love this hash recipe because it's an easy way to fuel myself for long, hard days in the saddle. It's a combination of several of my favorite foods that just so happen to be tasty, quick, and filling. As an extra bonus, it's also really inexpensive to make!"

1 For the Chili Spice Blend: In a small bowl, combine the garlic powder, paprika, and chili powder and set aside.

2 For the Hash: Preheat the oven to 400°F. Line a baking sheet with parchment paper and grease with cooking spray.

3 In a large bowl, combine the onion, sweet potatoes, bell pepper, and black beans. Drizzle with olive oil and sprinkle the spice blend on top. Toss to evenly coat. Spread the mixture onto the prepared baking sheet and season with salt and pepper. Bake for 35 to 40 minutes, tossing halfway through, until the sweet potatoes are golden and tender.

4 Remove from the oven and make six wells in the vegetable mixture. Crack one of the eggs into a small bowl and then carefully slide the egg into one of the wells. Repeat with the remaining eggs. Season with salt and pepper. Return to the oven and bake for 6 to 8 minutes, until the whites are set but the yolks are still runny.

5 Garnish with avocado and cilantro, and serve with hot sauce and lime wedges.

PREP TIME// 15 minutes
COOK TIME// 50 minutes
SERVES// 4 to 6

Chili Spice Blend

½ teaspoon garlic powder

1 teaspoon sweet paprika

½ teaspoon chili powder

Hash

Olive oil cooking spray, for greasing

½ large red onion, roughly chopped

2 large sweet potatoes, peeled and cut into 1-inch cubes (3 to 4 cups)

1 green bell pepper, cored, seeded, and cut into 1-inch pieces

1 (15-ounce) can black beans, drained, rinsed, and patted dry

2 tablespoons extra-virgin olive oil

6 large eggs

Sea salt and freshly ground black pepper to taste

1 avocado, pitted, peeled, and diced, to garnish

¼ cup chopped fresh cilantro, to garnish

Hot sauce, to serve

Lime wedges, to serve

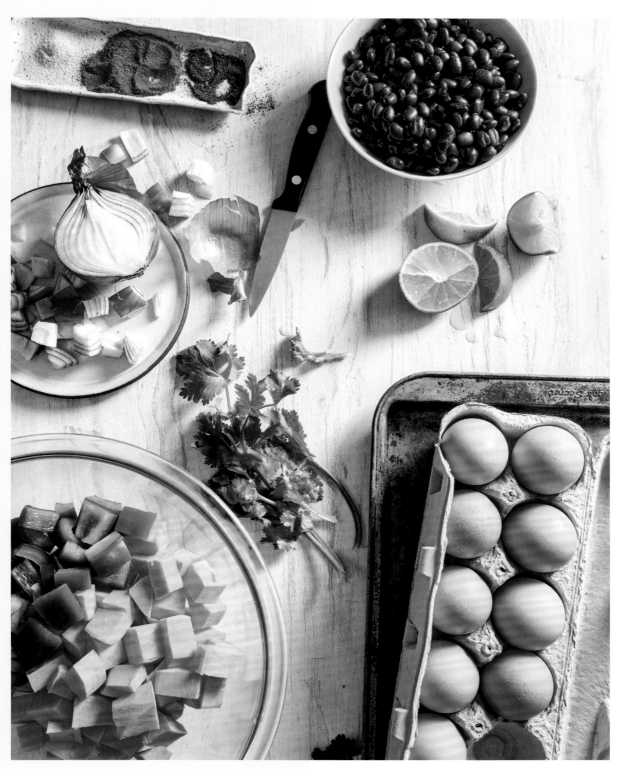

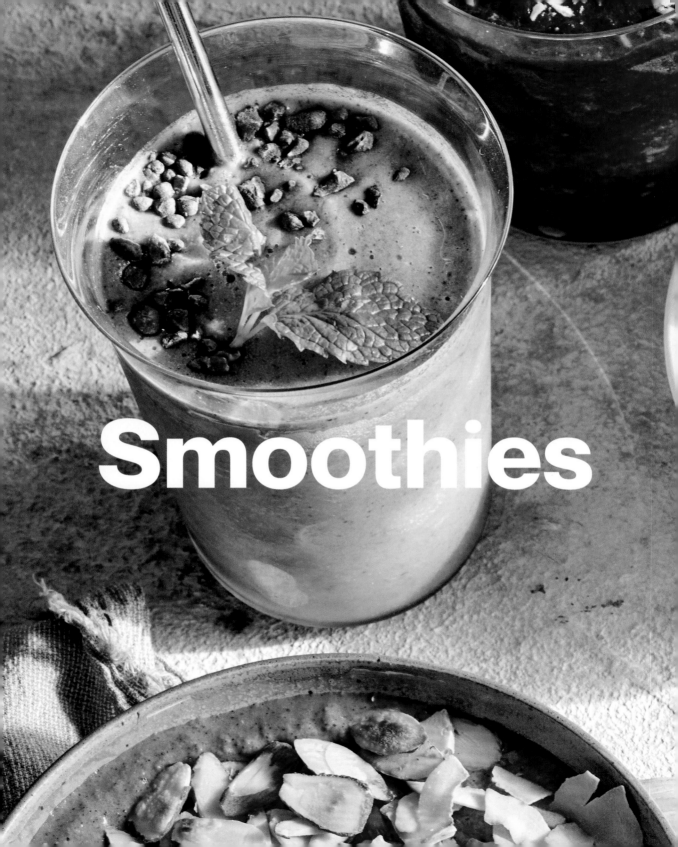

Smoothies

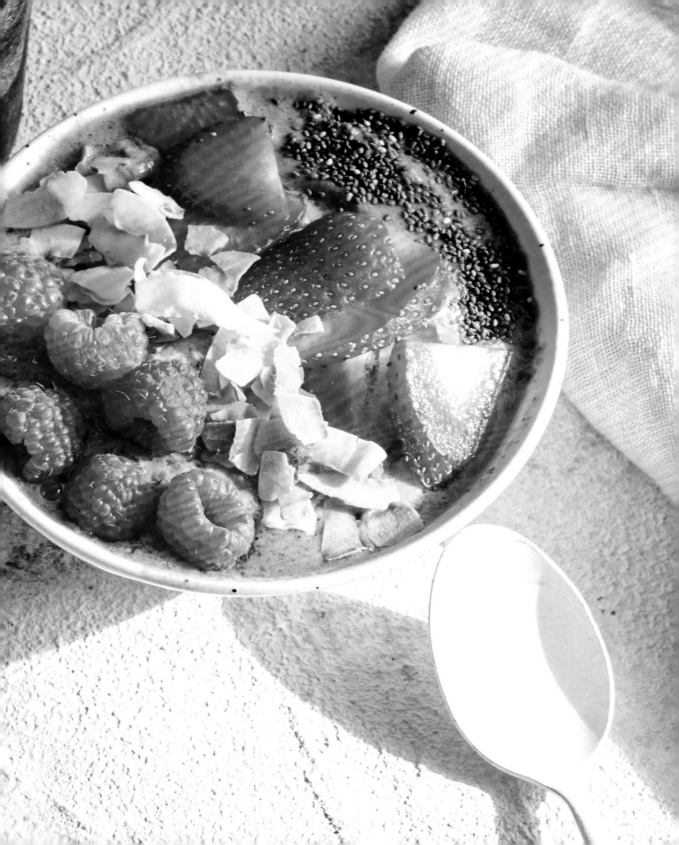

Smoothies are always fun to experiment with in the kitchen. Pick your most loved fruit, vegetables, nut butters, and flavor boosters for a drink that's nutritious and filling any time of day. No fancy blender needed—a good smoothie can be made with any standard machine. Often, I'm asked questions about how to build the ideal nutrient-dense smoothie as well as secrets to blending a smoothie correctly for the perfect consistency. Here are my tips and tricks.

The Six Components of a Smoothie

Every smoothie should always have a liquid, fruit, vegetable, protein, and fat. Flavor boosters are a nice addition but optional. All the smoothies and smoothie bowls I've included in this chapter have at least one type of vegetable, which is a pretty awesome way to add more veggie nutrients into your daily routine!

Liquid: Be sure to check the label for unsweetened nut and oat milks. You'd be surprised by how many brands sneak in sweeteners. Coconut water is also a refreshing and hydrating liquid option.

Fruit: Besides being delicious, fruit is the key to naturally sweeten a smoothie. I usually always stick to frozen fruit since it helps with thickening the smoothie, for a great consistency. It's also so easy to store frozen fruit for a month or two. If you have any bananas or other fruits that are too ripe to eat, place in an even layer inside a zip-top bag (laying them as flat as possible) in the freezer—they are perfect for smoothies. Additionally, rather than sweetening my smoothies with refined sugar, honey, or maple syrup, I use Medjool dates. This whole fruit sweetener provides extra fiber and nutrients and won't give you a sugar rush pre- or post-workout.

Vegetables: Pick your favorite greens or veggies here. I always try to focus on which veggies are in season to add to my smoothies. With greens, I use whatever I already have on hand in my refrigerator for the week. I also keep frozen kale and spinach in my freezer to add when I'm in a pinch, like coming home from a long week of traveling. Adding frozen cruciferous veggies, like frozen riced cauliflower or even frozen broccoli, adds bulk to the smoothie with mild flavor. Lastly, veggie purees like pumpkin puree or sweet potato puree may not initially come to mind when making a smoothie, but they help with creating an extra-smooth texture as well as a rich flavor to any smoothie base.

Protein Powder: Protein can be an optional ingredient if you are planning to add nut butter (which falls under the fat category but also provides protein) to your smoothie. When adding protein powder, look for a non-GMO plant-based protein powder that has at least 15 grams of protein per serving. Check what it's sweetened with—I opt for stevia sweetened or unsweetened. I use unflavored protein powder for smoothies that have a lot of flavor boosters like spices, mint, extracts, fresh ginger, or coffee. Vanilla and chocolate protein powders are great for smoothies when you want to enhance a vanilla or chocolate flavor. If you are adding vanilla protein powder, there's no need to add vanilla extract to the smoothie, and with chocolate protein powder, you can decrease the amount of cocoa powder to your preference.

Fat: Fat is an ingredient often forgotten in smoothies, but it's essential. Fat helps balance the flavor and texture in the smoothie, but more important, it keeps you full since it takes longer to digest. Fat is also important to consume pre- and post-workout as a fuel source for your body. Look for your preferred unsweetened natural nut butters when adding fat, but remember: the only ingredient in a nut butter should be nuts! Avocado and tahini are two savory options for healthy fats. Raw nuts are great as well if you desire some texture in the smoothie.

Flavor Boosters: This is where you get to have a lot of fun with your smoothie! Try adding extracts, spices, fresh herbs, fresh ginger, coffee beans, and matcha to a smoothie to make it a unique theme and flavor. For herbs and extracts, try adding fresh mint, or vanilla, peppermint, or maple extracts. The world of spices can add so many things to the flavor of a smoothie. Cinnamon, nutmeg, and a pinch of cayenne are just a few I use. Fresh ginger and turmeric are two important roots for anti-inflammation and gut health that also add a fresh flavor. If you need a caffeine boost, add whole coffee beans, cold brew, maca root powder, matcha, or concentrated unsweetened tea.

How to Blend the Perfect Smoothie

We've all been there, the smoothie gets stuck in the blade and you're not sure what to do, or the texture isn't smooth and it's too thick or too watery. Smoothie blending is very easy with these tips!

- Blend your greens first! This creates liquid for the smoothie and doesn't leave you with little pieces of kale throughout.

- Add liquid second and make sure you have enough liquid. This is key to smoothie success. Definitely keep this in mind when making a smoothie bowl. A smoothie bowl uses much less liquid than you would think to make the mixture thick enough that it can hold the toppings. I usually start with ¼ cup liquid for a smoothie

bowl and work my way up from there until the consistency is just right.

- Add ice, only as needed, after all other ingredients are blended together. Adding ice will thicken the smoothie, but you may not need it at all if you are using a lot of frozen fruit or veggies.

Smoothie Guide

pick one from each category

1 LIQUID
Unsweetened Almond Milk
Unsweetened Coconut Milk
Unsweetened Oat Milk
Coconut Water
Water

2 FRUIT
Banana
Berries
Mango
Dates
Cherries
Pineapple

3 VEGETABLE
Kale
Spinach
Cauliflower
Zucchini
Pumpkin Puree

4 PROTEIN
Protein Powder—Vega, Garden of Life

5 FAT
Nut Butter
Avocado
Tahini
Nuts

6 FLAVOR BOOSTERS (OPTIONAL)
Fresh Mint
Ginger
Cinnamon
Nutmeg
Matcha Powder
Coffee Grounds

Pumpkin Pie Smoothie

PREP TIME// 5 minutes

SERVES// 1

½ cup pumpkin puree

1 tablespoon unsweetened natural almond butter

1 pitted Medjool date

½ teaspoon ground cinnamon

¼ teaspoon ground nutmeg

Pinch of ground cloves (optional)

½ teaspoon vanilla extract (only if using unflavored protein powder)

2 tablespoons unflavored or vanilla protein powder

1 cup unsweetened nut milk

4 to 6 ice cubes

Pumpkin puree is an ingredient I always have on hand in my pantry. This smoothie happens to highlight pumpkin puree for the fall season. It provides a healthy vegetable base rich in immune-boosting vitamin A and vitamin C as well as the classic flavor everyone loves.

In the carafe of a high-speed blender, blend the pumpkin puree, almond butter, date, cinnamon, nutmeg, cloves (if using), vanilla (if using), protein powder, and nut milk until smooth. Add ice cubes and blend until the desired consistency is reached.

TIP: Try using boiled sweet potato or butternut squash as a substitute for pumpkin puree—also delicious!

Energized Mocha Crunch Smoothie

PREP TIME// 5 minutes

SERVES// 1

1 cup unsweetened nut milk

1 cup packed baby spinach

1 frozen banana

1 to 2 tablespoons coffee beans

¼ cup old-fashioned rolled oats

1 tablespoon unsweetened natural almond butter

2 pitted Medjool dates

1 teaspoon vanilla extract (only if using unflavored protein powder)

2 tablespoons unflavored or vanilla protein powder

½ teaspoon ground cinnamon

1 tablespoon unsweetened cocoa powder or cacao powder

4 to 6 ice cubes

Coffee is one of my favorite flavors, so naturally I had to create a coffee smoothie. This smoothie has a nice caffeine boost, and the rolled oats provide both creaminess and a source of complex carbohydrates. The surprise "crunch" from the whole coffee beans was actually created mistakenly when an athlete used whole coffee beans instead of brewed coffee in the original recipe—it's been a hit ever since!

In the carafe of a high-speed blender, blend the nut milk and spinach until smooth. Add the banana, coffee beans, oats, almond butter, dates, vanilla (if using), protein powder, cinnamon, and cocoa powder and blend again until smooth. Add ice cubes and blend until the desired consistency is reached.

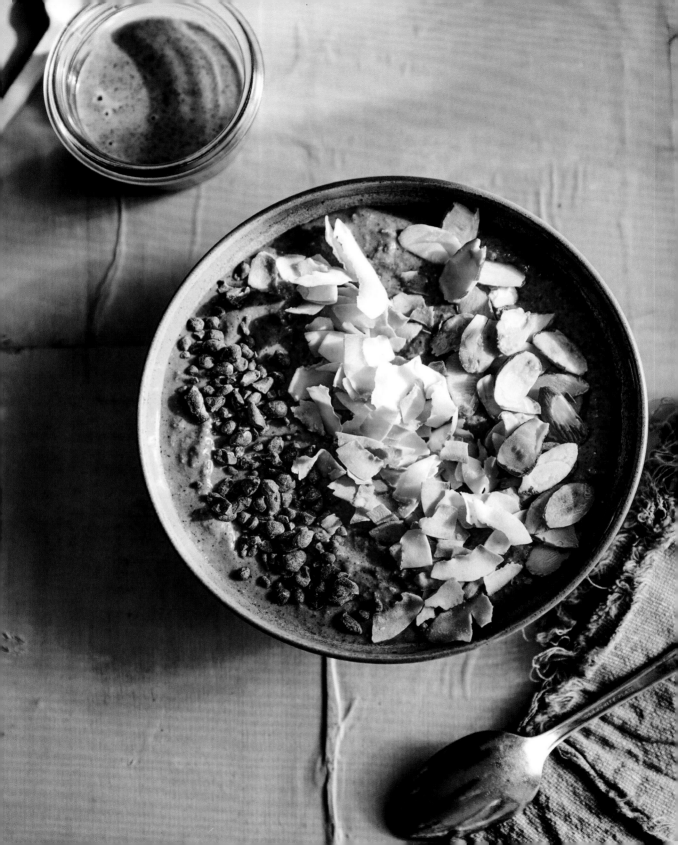

Chocolate Almond Smoothie Bowl

PREP TIME// 10 minutes

SERVES// 1

1 cup frozen riced cauliflower

½ cup unsweetened nut milk, plus additional if needed

1 to 2 tablespoons unsweetened natural almond butter

1 tablespoon cocoa powder

2 tablespoons chocolate, vanilla, or unsweetened protein powder

1 frozen banana

3 or 4 ice cubes

Toppings

1 tablespoon cacao nibs

2 tablespoons sliced almonds, toasted (see Note)

2 tablespoons unsweetened coconut flakes, toasted (see Note on page 76)

1 tablespoon unsweetened natural almond butter (thinned out with hot water if you desire a drizzle)

This smoothie bowl is for the chocolate lover who also loves crunch. The hidden surprise in the smoothie base is frozen riced cauliflower. I always make sure to have some of this in my freezer to use in smoothies because it adds a vegetable as well as some additional fiber that keeps me satisfied before or after a workout.

1   In the carafe of a high-speed blender, blend the cauliflower, nut milk, almond butter, cocoa powder, and protein powder until smooth. Add the banana and blend again until smooth, adding another tablespoon or two of nut milk if needed. Add ice cubes and blend until the desired consistency is reached—it should be much thicker than a normal smoothie.

2   Pour into a bowl and top with cacao nibs, almonds, coconut flakes, and almond butter.

NOTE: Toast the almonds until golden brown and fragrant.

Farmers' Market Smoothie

PREP TIME// 5 minutes

SERVES// 1

½ cup packed Swiss chard or baby spinach

½ medium zucchini, roughly chopped

1 cup frozen blackberries, plus additional to garnish

1 (1-inch) piece fresh ginger, peeled and grated

2 pitted Medjool dates

1 tablespoon ground flaxseed or hemp hearts

1 tablespoon fresh lemon juice

¼ avocado, pitted and peeled

1 cup unsweetened nut milk

4 to 6 ice cubes

TIP: When going to the farmers' market, I always bring my own bag or cooler bag in an effort to continue practicing sustainability. For similar reasons, if I know I'm going to cook a recipe in the next day or so, I try to buy the "ugly" produce to prevent it from being wasted (and it's often cheaper!).

Spending an afternoon at the farmers' market is something I always look forward to on the weekend. I buy all sorts of berries and freeze them to have farm-fresh smoothies all year-round. I love adding fresh greens and mild veggies, like zucchini, to my smoothies for additional vitamins and nutrients. I use avocado in this smoothie as a source of healthy fat that also adds a unique and delicious creamy texture.

In the carafe of a high-speed blender, blend the Swiss chard and zucchini until smooth. Add the blackberries, ginger, dates, flaxseed, lemon juice, avocado, and nut milk and blend again until smooth. Add ice cubes and blend until the desired consistency is reached. Garnish with blackberries.

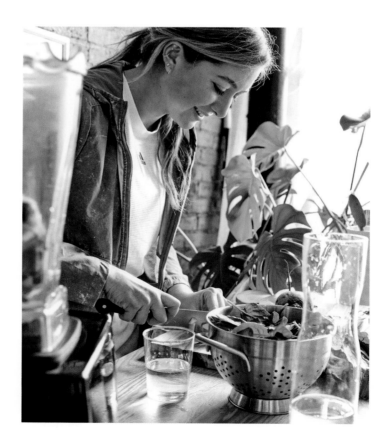

Tahini Date Smoothie

PREP TIME// 5 minutes +
15 minutes soaking

SERVES// 1

2 pitted Medjool dates, halved

Hot water (115°F to 120°F), to cover dates

½ cup frozen riced cauliflower

1 cup unsweetened nut milk

½ frozen banana

1 tablespoon tahini

1 teaspoon vanilla extract

¼ teaspoon ground cinnamon, plus additional to garnish

3 or 4 ice cubes

Optional Toppings

1 tablespoon cocoa powder

¼ cup old-fashioned rolled oats

1 tablespoon ground flaxseed

1 tablespoon hemp seed

I was inspired to make this smoothie as a Middle Eastern version of Mexican horchata, a creamy sweet cinnamon drink made from rice. This smoothie is lightly sweetened, rich with cinnamon, and has a hint of nutty flavor from the tahini. Plus, it's a great way to add extra vegetables and calcium to your daily routine.

1 In a small heatproof bowl, cover the dates with hot water and allow to soak for 15 minutes to soften. Drain and discard the liquid.

2 In the carafe of a high-speed blender, blend the cauliflower and nut milk until smooth. Add the softened dates, banana, tahini, vanilla, and cinnamon and blend again until smooth. Add ice cubes and blend until the desired consistency is reached.

3 Pour into a glass, dust with additional cinnamon, and add toppings, if desired.

Antioxidant Pink Smoothie Bowl

PREP TIME// 5 minutes

SERVES// 1

½ cup baby kale or your favorite green

¼ cup unsweetened nut milk

½ cup frozen strawberries

½ cup frozen raspberries

½ frozen banana

1 tablespoon unsweetened natural almond butter

1 pitted Medjool date

2 tablespoons unflavored or vanilla protein powder (optional)

4 or 5 ice cubes

Toppings

2 sliced strawberries

¼ cup fresh raspberries

2 tablespoons unsweetened coconut flakes, toasted (see Note)

1 teaspoon chia seeds

1 tablespoon unsweetened natural almond butter (optional)

Being creative with smoothie bowls is a fun way to begin the day. It's important with a smoothie bowl to use much less liquid than you would with a regular smoothie because the mixture needs to be thick enough to hold all the delicious toppings. This pink smoothie bowl is full of antioxidants like anthocyanins, ellagic acid, and resveratrol. Antioxidants help protect your cells from free radicals, which are molecules that can cause cell damage if they are too abundant.

1 In the carafe of a high-speed blender, blend the kale and nut milk until smooth. Add the strawberries, raspberries, banana, almond butter, date, and protein powder (if using) and blend again until smooth. Add ice cubes and blend until the desired consistency is reached—the mixture should be pretty thick.

2 Scrape the smoothie into a bowl and top with the sliced strawberries, raspberries, coconut flakes, and a sprinkle of chia seeds. Add a dollop of almond butter (if using) and serve.

NOTE: To toast the coconut flakes: In a small sauté pan, toast the coconut flakes over medium-low heat until lightly golden and fragrant, about 4 minutes. Remove from the pan and allow to cool.

TIP: When making a smoothie bowl, which requires much less liquid than a regular smoothie, I always start with ¼ cup liquid and work my way up from there until it's the consistency of a thick hummus.

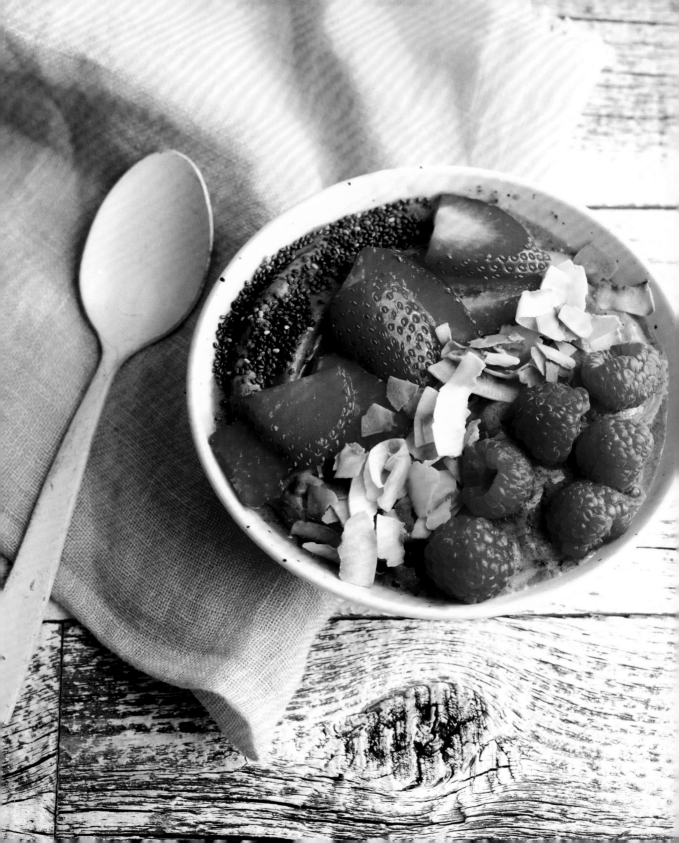

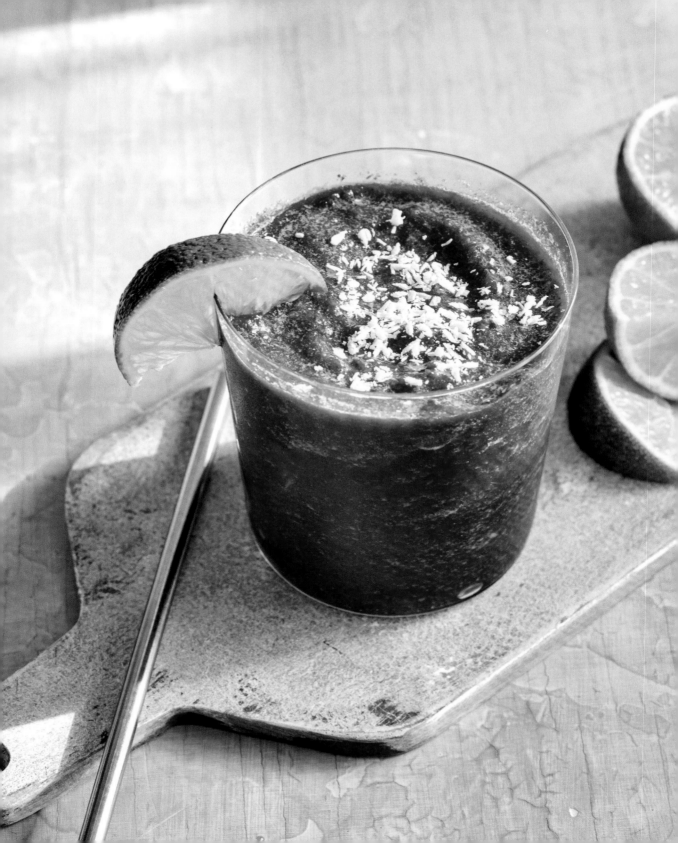

Anti-Inflammatory Beet Mango Smoothie

PREP TIME// 5 minutes

SERVES// 1

1 small beet, peeled and chopped (about ⅓ cup)

1 cup packed leafy greens, such as baby kale, spinach, Swiss chard, or romaine

1 (1-inch) piece fresh ginger, peeled and sliced

½ cup fresh or frozen mango

1 cup frozen cherries

1 tablespoon chia seeds

1 lime, juiced

1 cup coconut water

4 or 5 ice cubes

Lime wedge, for garnish

1 tablespoon unsweetened shredded coconut, to garnish

Raw beets in a smoothie may sound strange, but they're extremely delicious and refreshing for a post-workout recovery drink. Not only do beets have almost all the vitamins and minerals you need, but their natural nitrates have also been found to improve athletic performance. Nitrates are important because they help promote blood flow and energy production as well as possibly help with the negative effects of reduced oxygen availability that come with intense training.

In the carafe of a high-speed blender, blend the beet and greens until smooth. Add the ginger, mango, cherries, chia seeds, lime juice, and coconut water and blend again until smooth. Add ice cubes and blend until the desired consistency is reached. Garnish with a lime wedge and shredded coconut.

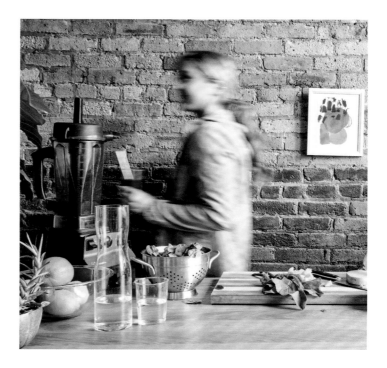

TIP: Always blend your greens first so they are incorporated nicely into the smoothie. This also allows for easy blending of the remaining ingredients after.

Green Ginger Smoothie Juice

PREP TIME// 5 minutes

SERVES// 1

2 cups packed leafy greens, such as baby kale, spinach, Swiss chard, or romaine

1 cup coconut water

1 (1-inch) piece fresh ginger, peeled and sliced

½ medium Granny Smith apple, peeled and cored

¼ cup fresh or frozen pineapple chunks

4½ teaspoons ground flaxseed

2 tablespoons tahini

3 tablespoons fresh lemon juice

4 to 6 ice cubes

If you love a juice, this smoothie is for you. I normally prefer smoothies to juices since you lose the natural vegetable fiber in juicing and oftentimes increase the natural sugars. This smoothie is different, though; it's lighter in texture to mimic a juice and uses the whole fruit and vegetable, ensuring you are maximizing the vitamins and nutrients.

In the carafe of a high-speed blender, blend the greens and coconut water until smooth. Add the ginger, apple, pineapple, flaxseed, tahini, and lemon juice and blend again until smooth. Add ice cubes and blend until the desired consistency is reached.

TIP: Fun twist! This smoothie is perfect to transform into a fruit- or veggie-based cocktail for an evening treat. Try adding a shot of vodka or tequila for a refreshing summer drink.

Molly Huddle's Ginger Cherry Smoothie

ATHLETE RECIPE: Molly Huddle is a two-time Olympian, multiple National Champion, and American record holder runner for the 5K, 10,000-meter, and half-marathon races. She lives and trains mainly in Rhode Island but also in Arizona.

"This is a smoothie I always have in my weekly routine; I probably make it about three times a week! It's one of my favorite ways to make an entirely plant-based drink that is full of vitamins and nutrients. Plus, I love that it keeps me hydrated and supplements my carbohydrate intake in a healthy way while I'm marathon training."

In the carafe of a high-speed blender, blend the rice milk and spinach until smooth. Add the cherries, ginger, banana, and protein powder (if using) and blend again until smooth. Add water if needed for consistency.

PREP TIME // 5 minutes

SERVES // 1

1 cup vanilla rice milk

½ cup baby spinach

½ cup frozen dark sweet cherries

1 (1-inch) piece fresh ginger, peeled

½ banana, peeled, or ½ avocado, peeled and pitted

2 tablespoons protein powder of choice (optional)

¼ cup water, if needed

Steph Bruce's Mint Chip Smoothie

ATHLETE RECIPE: Steph Bruce is a professional distance runner for HOKA NAZ Elite. She lives and trains in Flagstaff, Arizona, with her husband, Ben, and two boys. Lottie and Steph worked together on creating a nutrition strategy for the 2020 Olympic trials, where Lottie traveled to Flagstaff once a month to prepare food and work on dialing her nutrition. Steph was just nineteen seconds from making the Olympic team, finishing sixth.

"Truthfully, I've never been a fan of mint and chocolate together. It was actually Lottie who inspired me to make this smoothie when she made me a similar version in fall 2019. I must admit, I've been making this smoothie almost every day since. It's refreshing, with a hint of cocoa flavor and full of nutrients, perfect for post-workout recovery."

In the carafe of a high-speed blender, blend the almond milk and kale until smooth. Add the banana, almond butter, mint, cinnamon, and protein powder and blend again until smooth. Add ice cubes and blend until the desired consistency is reached. Stir in the cacao nibs. Garnish with mint leaves and additional cacao nibs.

NOTE: If you are using unflavored protein powder, add 1 teaspoon vanilla extract to this smoothie.

PREP TIME// 5 minutes
SERVES// 1

1 cup unsweetened almond milk

1 cup packed baby kale

1 frozen banana

1 tablespoon unsweetened natural almond butter

2 tablespoons fresh mint leaves, plus additional to garnish

Pinch of ground cinnamon

2 tablespoons vanilla or unflavored protein powder (see Note)

4 to 6 ice cubes

1 tablespoon cacao nibs, plus additional to garnish

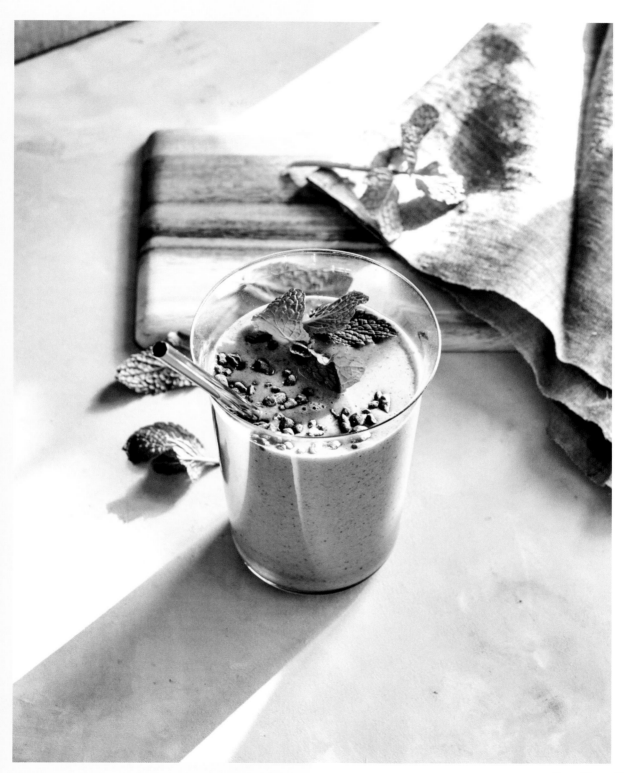

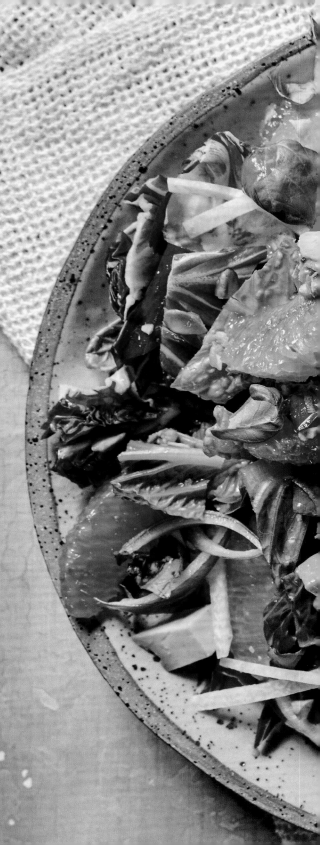

Bowls

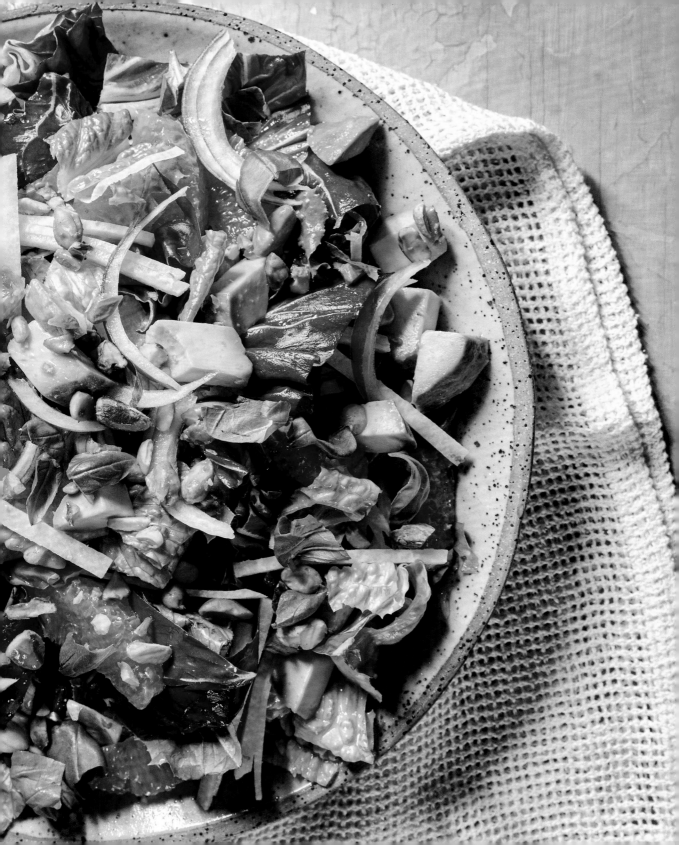

Bowls are the perfect meal: they often have a grain, veggies, protein, and delicious sauce, stock, or dressing to tie all the flavors together! Plus, they are easy to meal-prep for the week and take on the go. Bowls can be grain or salad based, or they can be a hearty stew. When I first started cooking, bowls were one of the first savory meals I would experiment with—they are simple to make but so creative, and they're pretty much always delicious!

In this chapter, I share some of my best bowls that are full of different textures and flavors. I think when creating a successful grain bowl, whether salad bowl or stew, it's important to first pick your favorite veggies, proteins, grains, and flavor enhancers, like nuts, spices, and sauces. Next, pick a theme. I chose a Mediterranean theme for my Falafel Slider Greek Salad Bowl (page 105), an Italian one for my Supergreen Pasta (page 112), and a Mexican-BBQ fusion for my BBQ Fajita Bowl (page 89). Choosing a theme helps me narrow down the toppings and flavor enhancers I want to use to make an easy recipe on the fly that is crazy flavorful. Check out my Flavor Guide (page 27) for more information on ingredients and spices to use for different flavor profiles.

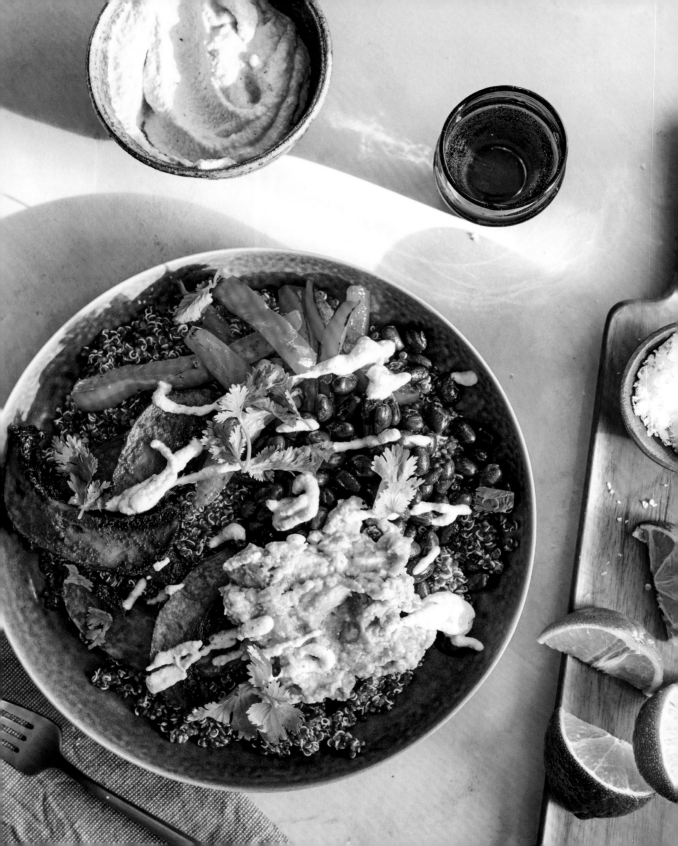

BBQ Fajita Bowl

PREP TIME// 15 minutes

COOK TIME// 30 minutes

SERVES// 4

Mushroom Bacon and Roasted Peppers

¼ cup avocado oil

2 tablespoons apple cider vinegar

2 tablespoons liquid aminos
(I like Bragg)

1½ teaspoons smoked paprika

½ teaspoon ground cumin

¼ teaspoon garlic powder

1 tablespoon tomato paste

2 portabella mushrooms, stems
removed, and sliced ¼-inch thick

2 red bell peppers, cored, seeded,
and thinly sliced

Sea salt and freshly ground black
pepper to taste

Quinoa Bowl

1½ cups red quinoa, rinsed

1 (15-ounce) can black beans, drained,
and rinsed

1 avocado, pitted, peeled, and mashed

Sea salt and freshly ground black
pepper to taste

¼ cup fresh cilantro leaves, to garnish

1 lime, cut into wedges, to serve

1 recipe Vegan Ranch Dressing
(page 237), to serve

Grain bowls are always one of my favorite meals because you can be so creative. This one happens to be inspired by my love of Mexican flavors. The mushroom bacon is the highlight in this bowl. It has a smoky spice rub to mimic carnitas. These mushrooms are also a great addition to any sandwich or salad.

1 **For the Mushroom Bacon and Roasted Peppers:** Preheat the oven to 400°F. Line two rimmed baking sheets with parchment paper.

2 In a small bowl, combine 2 tablespoons of the avocado oil, the vinegar, liquid aminos, paprika, cumin, garlic powder, and tomato paste. Brush over both sides of the mushrooms several times. Place the mushrooms on one of the prepared baking sheets.

3 In a large bowl, toss the bell peppers with the remaining 2 tablespoons avocado oil and season with salt and pepper. Place on the second prepared baking sheet. Roast the mushrooms on the top rack of the oven and the peppers on the bottom. Allow to cook for 20 to 25 minutes, or until the mushrooms are crispy and fragrant and the peppers are lightly golden.

4 **For the Quinoa Bowl:** Cook the quinoa according to the package instructions. Divide the quinoa among four bowls. Top with the mushroom bacon, roasted peppers, black beans, and mashed avocado. Season the avocado in each bowl with a pinch of salt and pepper and then sprinkle the cilantro leaves on top. Serve with lime wedges and a drizzle of dressing.

Vegan Chickpea Kale Caesar

PREP TIME// 15 minutes +
15 minutes soaking

COOK TIME// 30 minutes

SERVES// 4

Vegan Caesar Dressing

½ cup raw cashews

Hot water (115°F to 120°F), to cover cashews, plus additional ¼ cup

1 teaspoon Dijon mustard

1 tablespoon capers, drained

2 tablespoons nutritional yeast

3 tablespoons fresh lemon juice

2 garlic cloves

¼ cup extra-virgin olive oil

Sea salt and freshly ground black pepper to taste

Kale Salad

1 (15-ounce) can chickpeas, drained and rinsed

2 tablespoons avocado oil

1 teaspoon dried thyme

Sea salt and freshly ground black pepper to taste

2 (12-ounce) bunches of lacinato kale, stems removed, and thinly sliced

1 lemon, zested

¼ cup Almond Parmesan (page 241)

When I switched to a plant-based diet, it was difficult to find a Caesar salad recipe that had the same flavor and tang you would find in a traditional Caesar dressing, so I developed a recipe to make it deliciously vegan. This cashew-based dressing is cheesy from the nutritional yeast as well as briny from the capers. Plus, the addition of crunchy chickpeas mimics croutons and adds a protein boost. This recipe is an all-around winner for a simple weekday lunch or dinner with friends.

1 **For the Vegan Caesar Dressing:** In a small heatproof bowl, cover the cashews with hot water and allow to soak for 15 minutes to soften. Drain and discard the liquid.

2 Transfer the softened cashews to the carafe of a high-speed blender. Add the mustard, capers, nutritional yeast, lemon juice, garlic, olive oil, and the ¼ cup hot water and blend until smooth. Season with salt and pepper to taste. Set aside.

3 **For the Kale Salad:** Preheat the oven to 425°F. Line a baking sheet with parchment paper.

4 Pat the chickpeas very dry. Place on the prepared baking sheet and toss with the avocado oil, and thyme and season with salt and pepper. Allow to roast for 25 to 30 minutes, tossing halfway through, until crispy. Remove from the oven and allow to cool.

5 Toss the kale with ½ cup of the dressing and allow to marinate for 10 minutes. Add additional dressing if you like it heavier or save the rest in the refrigerator for a salad the next day. Divide among four plates and top with chickpeas, lemon zest, and the "parm."

TIP: Because kale is such a sturdy green, this salad is great the next day. The dressing helps wilt the kale over time and make it tender. No need to worry about soggy greens if you dress this salad several hours before serving!

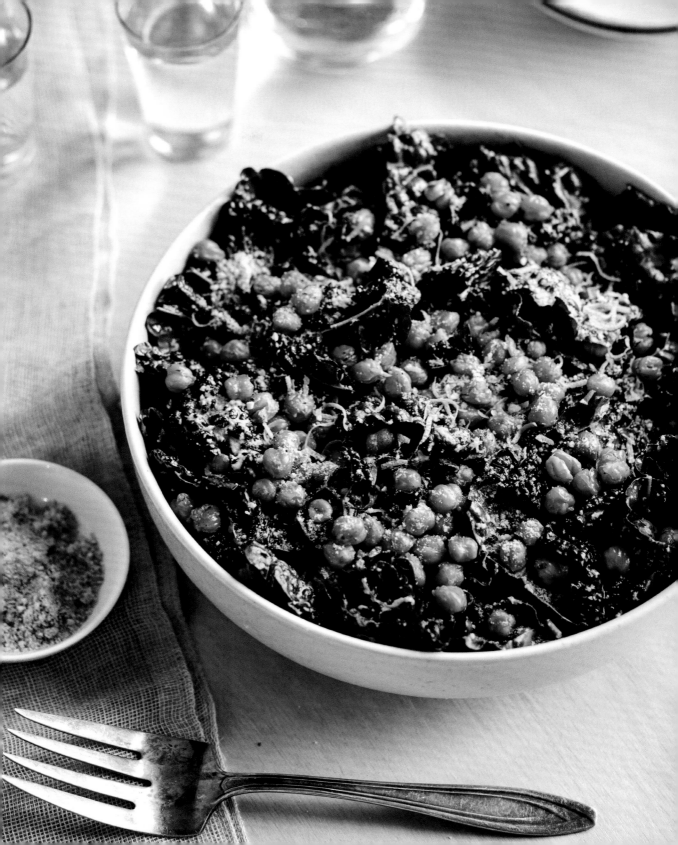

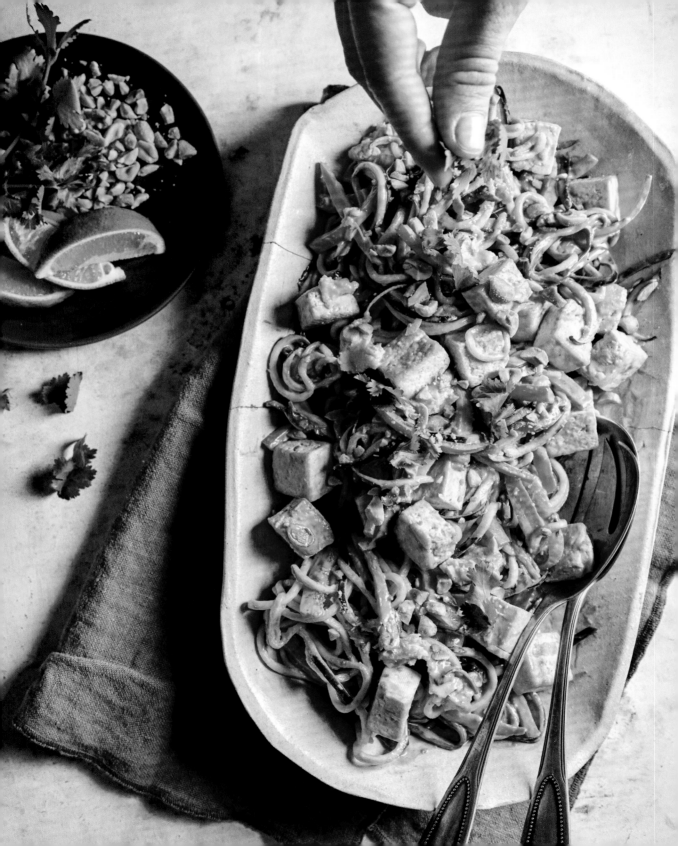

Spicy Peanut Tofu Pad Thai

PREP TIME// 20 minutes +
10 minutes draining
COOK TIME// 30 minutes
SERVES// 4

Pad Thai Sauce

½ cup unsweetened natural creamy
peanut butter

¼ cup fresh lime or lemon juice

¼ cup liquid aminos (I like Bragg)

2 tablespoons to ¼ cup sriracha
(depending on how spicy you like it!)

1 tablespoon toasted sesame oil

Noodle Bowl

1 (12-ounce) package firm tofu, drained

2 tablespoons avocado oil, plus
additional as needed

Sea salt to taste

Bunch of scallions (white and light
green parts), finely chopped

2 garlic cloves, minced

1 (1-inch) piece of ginger, peeled
and grated

4 cups shredded red cabbage

4 medium carrots, sliced into
matchsticks

1 red bell pepper, cored, seeded, and
thinly sliced into strips

1 pound zucchini, spiralized
(about 4 cups)

4 large eggs, lightly beaten

¼ cup chopped fresh cilantro,
to garnish

¼ cup roasted and salted peanuts,
chopped, to garnish

2 limes, cut into wedges, to serve

If you love a good homemade peanut sauce, this pad Thai will be at the top of your recipe list. What I love about this recipe is it's made entirely of veggies! I used red cabbage and zucchini noodles as the base for the delicious peanut sauce. I also added scrambled eggs for additional protein, but feel free to omit for a vegan version. Additionally, if you are looking for a heartier bite, try adding brown rice pad Thai noodles.

1 **For the Pad Thai Sauce:** In a small bowl, whisk together the peanut butter, lime juice, liquid aminos, sriracha, and sesame oil. Set aside.

2 **For the Noodle Bowl:** Line a plate with paper towels. Place the tofu on top and place more paper towels on top of the tofu. Place a heavy pan on top of the tofu and allow the tofu to drain of excess liquid for 10 minutes. Pat very dry and cut the tofu into 1-inch cubes.

3 In a large nonstick sauté pan, heat the avocado oil over medium-high heat. Add the tofu and allow to cook for 8 to 10 minutes, until golden on all sides. Season with salt and remove to a plate.

4 Add more oil if the pan is nearly dry, then add half of the scallions, the garlic, and ginger. Cook for a minute until fragrant. Add the cabbage, carrots, and bell pepper and cook for another 6 to 7 minutes, until softened. Add the zucchini noodles and cook another 5 minutes, or until wilted but still with some texture. Season with salt.

5 Move the vegetables to one side of the pan to make a well for the eggs. Add the eggs and stir gently, allowing them to begin to set. Once small curds have formed, stir throughout the vegetable mixture.

6 Add the pad Thai sauce, cooked tofu, and the remaining scallions to the vegetable mixture. Toss to evenly coat. Season with more salt, if desired.

7 Divide pad Thai into four bowls and garnish with chopped cilantro and peanuts. Serve with lime wedges.

Southwestern Vegetable Slow Cooker Chili

PREP TIME// 10 minutes

COOK TIME// 5 minutes +
4 to 8 hours slow cooking

SERVES// 4

Chili

2 tablespoons avocado oil

1 medium yellow onion, diced

3 garlic cloves, minced

2 tablespoons tomato paste

2 tablespoons chili powder

2 teaspoons ground cumin

1 teaspoon smoked paprika

Pinch of cayenne pepper (optional)

Sea salt and freshly ground black
pepper to taste

1 red bell pepper, cored, seeded,
and diced

1 (15-ounce) can fire-roasted tomatoes

1 (15-ounce) can crushed tomatoes

9 ounces butternut squash, peeled,
seeded, and cut into ½-inch pieces
(about 2 cups)

1 (15-ounce) can black beans, drained
and rinsed

1 (15-ounce) can chickpeas, drained
and rinsed

½ cup water

Sea salt and freshly ground black
pepper to taste

Toppings

1 avocado, peeled, pitted, and diced

¼ cup fresh cilantro leaves

½ bunch scallions (white and green
parts), thinly sliced

Chili is the perfect meal for my slow cooker especially on a weekday when I know I won't have time to make dinner. This chili takes minimal prep time in the morning, and by the evening you have a delicious stew waiting for you at home. I serve this chili with my Farro Corn Bread (page 154).

1 For the Chili: In a large sauté pan, heat the avocado oil over medium-high heat. Add the onion and garlic and cook about 4 minutes, or until softened. Add the tomato paste, chili powder, cumin, paprika, and cayenne (if using). Season with salt and pepper and cook for an additional minute until fragrant.

2 Transfer the spiced onion mixture to the bowl of a 6-quart slow cooker and add the bell pepper, fire-roasted tomatoes, crushed tomatoes, squash, black beans, chickpeas, and water. Season with salt and pepper. Cover and set on low for 8 hours or high for 4 hours, until the squash is tender and the flavors have melded. Top with avocado, cilantro leaves, and scallions.

TIP: If you want to cook the chili on the stovetop, simmer for 40 to 45 minutes, stirring occasionally, with an additional 3 to 4 cups of water until the squash is tender, flavors have combined, and chili is thickened and fragrant.

Roasted Carrot-Kabocha Soup

with Spiced Pumpkin Seeds

PREP TIME// 20 minutes

COOK TIME// 50 minutes

SERVES// 4

Spiced Pumpkin Seeds

1 tablespoon avocado oil

½ cup raw pumpkin seeds

½ teaspoon chili powder

Sea salt to taste

Carrot-Kabocha Soup

1 small kabocha squash
(about 2 pounds), halved and seeded

¼ cup avocado oil

Sea salt and freshly ground black
pepper to taste

3 medium carrots, cut into
1-inch pieces

1 medium yellow onion, sliced

3 garlic cloves, crushed

½ teaspoon ground coriander

¼ teaspoon ground cinnamon

4 cups low-sodium vegetable stock

½ cup light coconut milk, well shaken,
plus additional to garnish

This is the first recipe I ever published on my blog and it's still one of my top winter soup recipes. I make a big batch in the fall and keep it in the freezer through the winter. I like using kabocha squash here because it's so flavorful and creamy, but it's also a great source of beta-carotene, which is converted into vitamin A for skin and eye health. Best of all, you can eat the kabocha squash skin, so no need to peel!

1 **For the Spiced Pumpkin Seeds:** In a small sauté pan, heat the avocado oil over medium-low heat. Add the pumpkin seeds, chili powder, and salt and allow to toast for 5 to 6 minutes, until golden and fragrant. Allow to cool before serving. Store in an airtight container at room temperature for up to 1 month.

2 **For the Carrot-Kabocha Soup:** Preheat the oven to 400°F. Line two baking sheets with parchment paper.

3 Drizzle the insides of the squash with 2 tablespoons of the avocado oil and season with salt and pepper. Place cut side down onto the first prepared baking sheet.

4 Toss the carrots, onion, garlic, coriander, and cinnamon with the remaining 2 tablespoons oil and season with salt and pepper. Place on the second prepared baking sheet. Roast the squash and carrots for 35 to 40 minutes, until the squash is tender and the carrots and onion are golden. Allow to cool slightly. Cut the squash into 1- to 2-inch pieces.

5 Transfer the squash to the carafe of a high-speed blender, add the carrot-onion mixture, and blend until smooth. Add half the stock and blend until very smooth. Transfer to a large pot, then add the remaining stock. Place the pot over medium-low heat and add the coconut milk. Stir to combine and heat until warmed through. Season with salt and pepper as needed. If the soup is thicker than you like, stir in water as needed to adjust consistency. Garnish with a drizzle of coconut milk and the spiced pumpkin seeds.

Thai Crunch Salad

PREP TIME// 15 minutes +
10 minutes marinating

SERVES// 4

Garlicky Peanut Ginger Soy Dressing

2 tablespoons rice wine vinegar

1 to 2 tablespoons apple cider vinegar

2 tablespoons liquid aminos (I like Bragg)

2 tablespoons fresh lime juice

1 tablespoon unsweetened natural creamy peanut butter

1 (2-inch) piece of ginger, peeled and grated

2 garlic cloves, grated

Pinch of red chili flakes (optional)

¼ cup avocado oil

Sea salt to taste

Thai Salad

2 cups shredded red cabbage

2 cups shredded Napa or green cabbage

1 red bell pepper, cored, seeded, and thinly sliced

½ bunch of scallions (white and light green parts), thinly sliced

½ cup fresh cilantro leaves

½ cup roasted unsalted peanuts, chopped

2 tablespoons toasted sesame seeds

This salad is full of colorful texture and crunch starting with the cabbage and red bell pepper at the base all the way to the peanuts and sesame seeds as the garnish. The delicious peanut dressing, with hints of soy, ginger, garlic, lime, and spice, brings all the flavors together.

1 **For the Garlicky Peanut Ginger Soy Dressing:** Whisk together the rice wine vinegar, apple cider vinegar, liquid aminos, lime juice, peanut butter, ginger, garlic, and chili flakes (if using). While whisking, slowly add in the avocado oil. Season with salt and set aside.

2 **For the Thai Salad:** In a large bowl, combine the red cabbage, Napa cabbage, bell pepper, scallions, and cilantro leaves. Drizzle the dressing over the mixed salad and toss to combine. Sprinkle with peanuts and sesame seeds. Allow the salad to marinate at least 10 minutes before eating (waiting longer is better for the flavors to meld and lettuce to soften!).

TIP: Marinate this salad with the dressing a couple hours in advance and store in the refrigerator for an even more peanut ginger flavor.

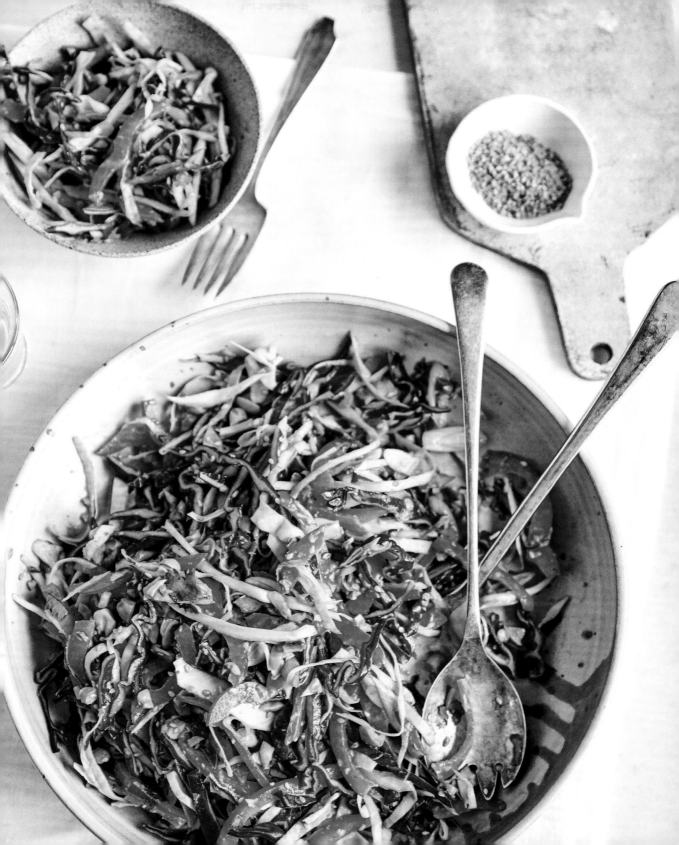

Soba Noodle Bowl

with Tahini and Tofu

PREP TIME// 25 minutes +
35 minutes draining + marinating
(up to overnight)
COOK TIME// 20 minutes
SERVES// 4

Marinated Tofu

1 (12-ounce) container firm tofu, drained

¼ cup liquid aminos (I like Bragg)

¼ cup rice wine vinegar

1 tablespoon apple cider vinegar

1 tablespoon toasted sesame oil

1 to 2 limes, juiced

Tahini Ginger Sauce

2 scallions (white and green parts), cut into 1-inch pieces

3 garlic cloves

1 (2-inch) piece of ginger, peeled and roughly chopped

⅓ cup tahini, well stirred

¼ cup liquid aminos (I like Bragg)

¼ cup rice wine vinegar

2 tablespoons toasted sesame oil

1 tablespoon apple cider vinegar

¼ teaspoon red chili flakes

When I'm craving a comforting noodle bowl, I turn to soba noodles, which are made from buckwheat flour. These noodles are rich in protein and fiber as well as manganese, which is good for glucose metabolism, and thiamin, which helps with cell function and growth. The noodles have a nutty flavor and pair great with the spicy and tangy Tahini Ginger Sauce. The seared tofu on top has a hint of lime and soy to make a bowl full of vibrant flavors.

1 **For the Marinated Tofu:** Line a plate with paper towels. Place the tofu on top of the paper towels and place more paper towels on top of the tofu. Place a heavy pan on top of the tofu and allow the tofu to drain of excess liquid for 10 minutes.

2 Meanwhile, in a medium bowl, combine the liquid aminos, rice wine vinegar, apple cider vinegar, sesame oil, and lime juice.

3 Once the tofu has drained, pat dry and cut into 1-inch cubes. Place in the bowl with the marinade, cover, and allow to marinate for at least 25 minutes or up to overnight in the refrigerator.

4 **For the Tahini Ginger Sauce:** In the bowl of a food processor fitted with the blade attachment, pulse the scallions, garlilc, ginger, tahini, liquid aminos, rice wine vinegar, toasted sesame oil, apple cider vinegar, and chili flakes until a smooth sauce forms. Scrape into a large bowl and set aside.

5 **For the Soba Noodle Bowl:** Bring a large pot of salted water to a boil.

6 In a large nonstick sauté pan, heat 1 tablespoon of the avocado oil over medium-high heat. Add the snow peas, bok choy, and cabbage and cook for 4 to 6 minutes, until just tender and wilted. Season with salt. Transfer to the bowl with the tahini ginger sauce and set aside.

Soba Noodle Bowl

Sea salt to taste

3 tablespoons avocado oil

1 cup snow peas, halved

2 heads of baby bok choy,
cut into 1-inch pieces

1 cup shredded red cabbage

1 (8-ounce) package soba noodles

1 tablespoon toasted sesame seeds,
to garnish

¼ cup chopped fresh cilantro,
to garnish

1 lime, cut into wedges, to serve

7 Pour the remaining 2 tablespoons oil into the same sauté pan. Add the tofu and marinade to the pan and cook for 8 to 10 minutes, until lightly golden (the marinade will reduce and evaporate, allowing the tofu to brown). Remove to a plate lined with paper towels.

8 Cook the soba noodles according to the package instructions. Drain the noodles, then immediately add to the large bowl with the cooked vegetables and the tahini ginger sauce. Toss well to combine. Divide the noodles among four bowls and top with the tofu. Garnish with sesame seeds and cilantro. Serve with lime wedges.

TIP: Be sure to look at the label and find a soba noodle that is made from 100% buckwheat flour since some brands use a buckwheat flour blend with fillers. You can prep all the ingredients for this recipe in advance, just cook the soba noodles right before serving since they get gummy after sitting for a while.

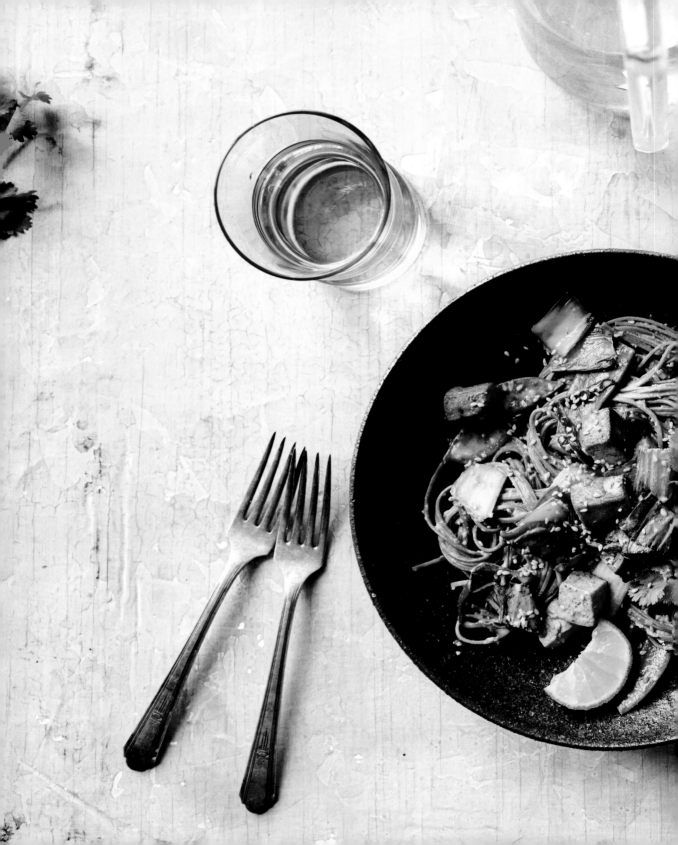

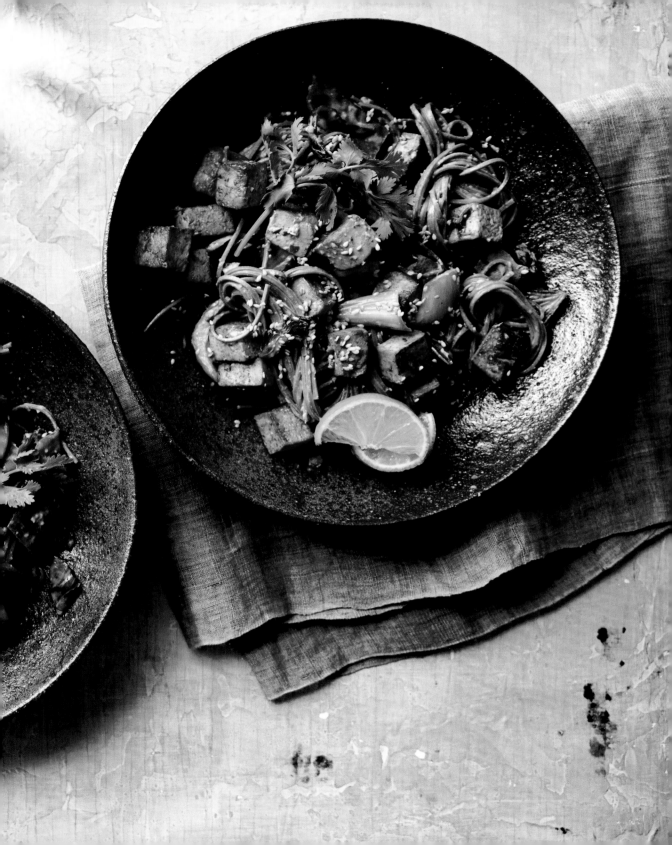

Pasta with Vodka Cream Sauce

PREP TIME// 5 minutes
COOK TIME// 15 minutes
SERVES// 4

Cashew Cream

1 cup raw cashews

½ cup hot water (115°F to 120°F)

Sea salt to taste

Pasta

Sea salt to taste

2 tablespoons avocado oil

1 medium yellow onion, diced small

4 garlic cloves, minced

Freshly ground black pepper to taste

¼ cup vodka

2 cups tomato puree

1 (16-ounce) package brown rice spaghetti

½ cup chopped fresh basil, to garnish

The secret to this creamy pasta recipe is cashews. When blended with hot water, they make a smooth "cream" to mix into sauces. When I have pasta night, this vodka sauce is always my first choice. The flavor of the tomato sauce is decadent and slightly nutty with the cashews, and the basil gives a light and fresh finish.

1 **For the Cashew Cream:** In the carafe of a high-speed blender, blend the cashews and hot water until smooth. Season with salt. Remove to a bowl and set aside.

2 **For the Pasta:** Bring a large pot of salted water to a boil. In a large sauté pan, heat the avocado oil over medium-high heat. Add the onion and garlic and cook about 4 minutes, or until softened. Season with salt and pepper to taste.

3 Remove the pan from the heat and add the vodka. Return the pan to the heat, add the tomato puree, and stir to combine. Season again with salt and pepper. Bring to a simmer and allow to cook another 3 to 4 minutes, until slightly thickened.

4 Remove from the heat and stir in the cashew cream mixture until combined and creamy. Season with salt and pepper if necessary.

5 Cook the pasta according to the package instructions. Reserve ½ cup of the pasta water. Drain and lightly rinse the pasta and immediately toss with the sauce, adding pasta water to bind if necessary. Top with the chopped basil and serve.

TIP: If you have leftover pasta, don't throw it out! Use it in a pasta casserole the next night. Mix 1 or 2 lightly beaten large eggs into the cold noodles and bake in an 8 × 8-inch baking dish at 400°F for 25 to 30 minutes, until the noodles are lightly golden brown and crispy on top. It's delicious!

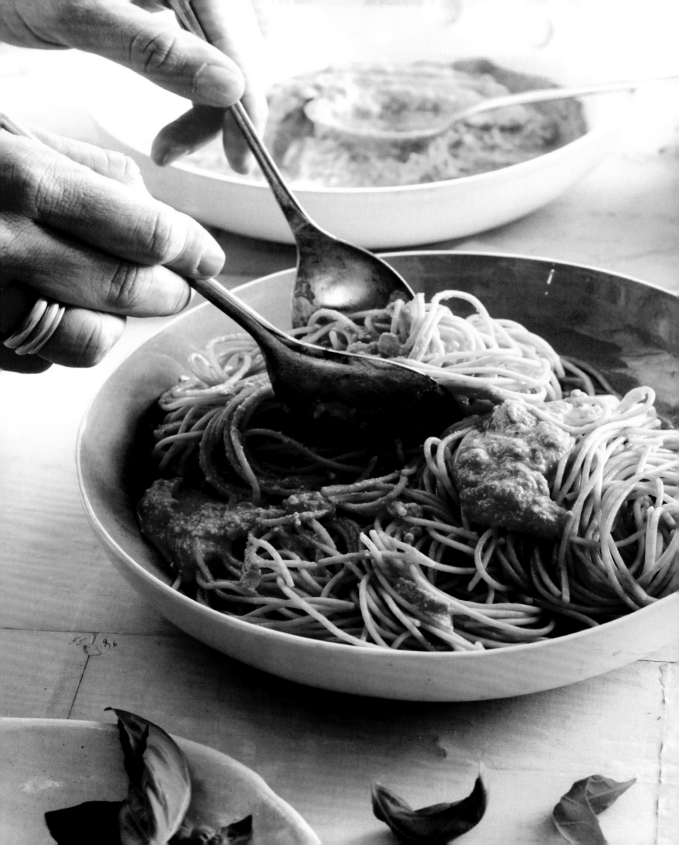

Broccoli Quinoa Salad

with Apples and Almonds

PREP TIME// 15 minutes

COOK TIME// 30 minutes

SERVES// 4

Dijon Vinaigrette

2 tablespoons Dijon mustard

3 tablespoons apple cider vinegar

1 teaspoon dried thyme

¼ cup extra-virgin olive oil

Sea salt and freshly ground black
pepper to taste

Quinoa Salad

2 cups broccoli florets

¼ cup avocado oil

Sea salt and freshly ground black
pepper to taste

1 small yellow onion, diced

2 garlic cloves, minced

1¼ cups quinoa, rinsed

4 cups water

⅓ cup chopped fresh flat-leaf parsley

1 large Honeycrisp apple, cored
and chopped

⅓ cup golden raisins

½ cup sliced almonds, toasted
(see Note)

This salad is similar to a grain bowl, with the ingredients tossed together instead of assembled in individual piles. It's a crowd-pleaser that's always requested for barbecues and picnics. My formula for a flavorful foolproof grain salad involves choosing a whole grain, a roasted veggie or fresh green, a dried fruit or nut, and a surprise ingredient like apple or berries, and then I toss everything together with a light dressing. It's a new and delicious recipe every time.

1 **For the Dijon Vinaigrette:** In a small bowl, whisk together the mustard, vinegar, and thyme. While whisking, slowly stream in the olive oil. Season with salt and pepper. Set aside.

2 **For the Quinoa Salad:** Preheat the oven to 400°F. Line a baking sheet with parchment paper.

3 Place the broccoli onto the prepared baking sheet and toss with 2 tablespoons of the avocado oil. Season with salt and pepper. Roast for 25 to 30 minutes, tossing halfway through, until tender with browned edges.

4 Meanwhile, in a medium saucepan, heat the remaining 2 tablespoons oil over medium-high heat. Add the onion and garlic and cook about 4 minutes, or until softened. Add the quinoa and toast an additional minute. Season with salt and pepper. Add water, bring to a boil, then reduce the heat and allow to simmer for 10 to 12 minutes, until quinoa is cooked through.

5 Once the quinoa is cooked, remove from the heat and place the lid on top for 5 minutes. Then fluff with a fork and transfer to a large bowl. Add the roasted broccoli, parsley, apple, golden raisins, and almonds. Drizzle the vinaigrette over the salad and toss to combine. Season with additional salt and pepper if necessary and serve immediately.

NOTE: For toasting the almonds: Place the almonds in a dry small sauté pan over medium-low heat. Allow to toast until golden brown and fragrant, 3 to 5 minutes. Remove from the heat and allow to cool completely.

Falafel Slider Greek Salad Bowl

PREP TIME// 15 minutes

COOK TIME// 40 minutes

SERVES// 4

Falafel Sliders

2 (15-ounce) cans chickpeas, drained and rinsed

½ cup fresh flat-leaf parsley

¼ cup fresh cilantro

½ cup fresh mint

¼ cup fresh lemon juice

¼ cup ground flaxseed

Pinch of cayenne pepper (optional)

1 small red onion, cut into large pieces

3 garlic cloves

Sea salt to taste

Avocado oil cooking spray
(I use a Misto)

Greek Salad

2 heads of romaine, cored and chopped

2 cups thinly sliced red cabbage

1 English cucumber, thinly sliced into half-moons

1 cup cherry tomatoes, halved

¼ cup pitted Kalamata olives, chopped

¼ cup Quick-Pickled Red Onions (page 238)

1 recipe Lemon Tahini Dressing (page 239)

Growing up in a Middle Eastern family, falafel has always been a mealtime staple. I wanted to create my own version of falafel that's herby with lots of garlic and lemon flavor. I bake this falafel to avoid adding excess oil from frying and place it on top a Greek salad, for a bowl I always crave.

1 **For the Falafel Sliders:** Preheat the oven to 375°F. Line a baking sheet with parchment paper.

2 Dry the chickpeas well and place on the prepared baking sheet. Roast for 10 minutes to slightly dry out the chickpeas. Allow to cool.

3 In the bowl of a food processor fitted with the blade attachment, pulse the parsley, cilantro, mint, lemon juice, flaxseed, cayenne, onion, and garlic until finely chopped. Add the chickpeas, season with salt, and pulse until the mixture just comes together but chickpeas are still roughly chopped (not too smooth).

4 Remove the mixture from the food processor and shape into ten ¼-cup slider patties. Grease the same parchment with cooking spray. Place the sliders onto the prepared baking sheet and spray the tops with cooking spray. Bake for 30 minutes, flipping halfway through, until golden brown and cooked through.

5 **For the Greek Salad:** In a large bowl, toss together the romaine, cabbage, cucumber, tomatoes, olives, and pickled onions. Divide among four plates and top with a couple of falafel sliders. Drizzle with the dressing and serve. Store leftover sliders in an airtight container in the refrigerator for up to 4 days.

TIPS: For all-natural avocado oil spray, I always use a Misto. It allows me to choose the oil I want to use when I'm cooking.

You can also use dried chickpeas for this recipe. The recipe will need 3 cups soaked chickpeas. Just make sure to soak the dried chickpeas for 24 hours at room temperature until they are tender, then drain and rinse before using. You also don't need to dry them out in the oven for 10 minutes prior to food processing.

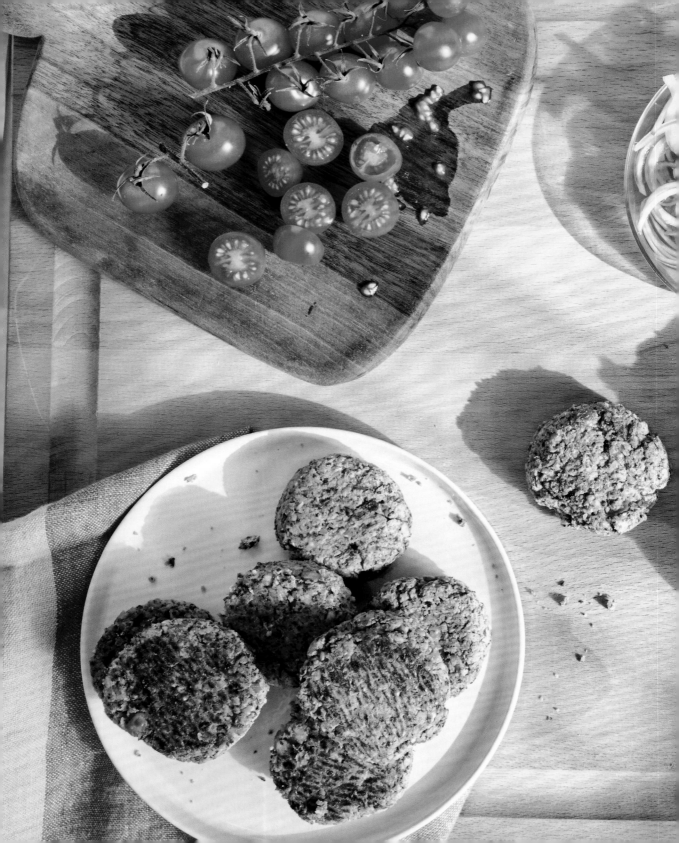

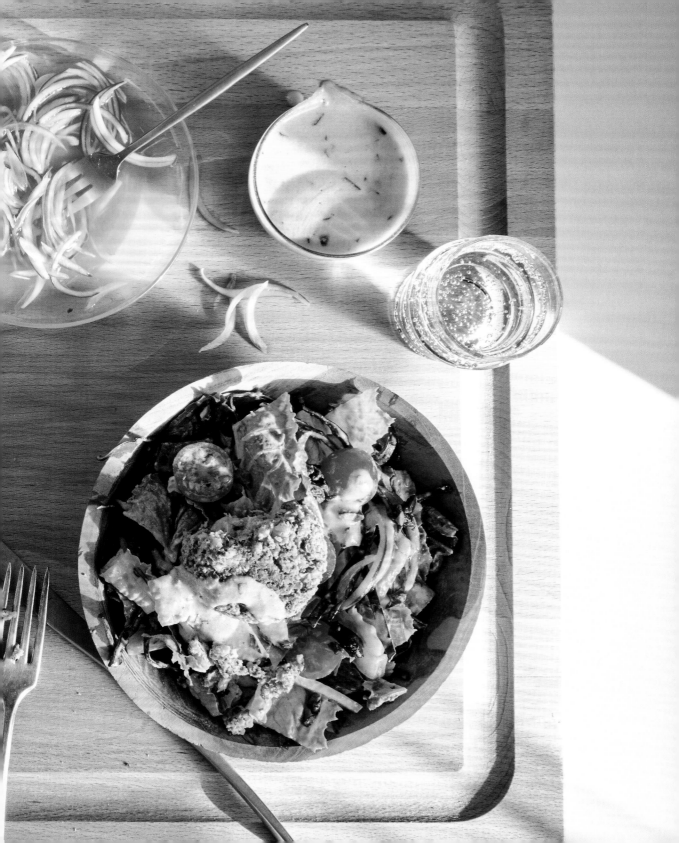

Jicama and Radicchio Chopped Salad

with Grapefruit

PREP TIME// 20 minutes

SERVES// 4

Citrus Basil Dressing

1 medium ruby grapefruit

2 limes, zested and juiced

¼ cup extra-virgin olive oil

Sea salt and freshly ground black pepper to taste

2 tablespoons roughly chopped fresh basil

Salad

Head of romaine, cored and chopped

½ head of radicchio, cored and chopped

4 ounces jicama, peeled and thinly sliced into matchsticks (about 1 cup)

1 avocado, pitted, peeled, and diced

½ red onion, thinly sliced

2 tablespoons roughly chopped fresh basil

¼ cup roasted and salted shelled pistachios, chopped, to garnish

Jicama is a unique ingredient that is readily available in more and more grocery stores. Often called a yam bean, it's high in fiber as well as inulin, which is a prebiotic good for gut health. It has great crunch and mild nutty flavor, so it complements fresh salads nicely. Pairing the jicama with grapefruit and radicchio makes for a tangy chopped salad full of texture. The avocado and pistachios add a creamy fat to balance the acid, and the basil brings a burst of freshness in the lime-based dressing.

1 **For the Citrus Basil Dressing:** Using a paring knife, cut off the top and bottom of the grapefruit so it can stand upright. Working from top to bottom, carefully cut the skin off the grapefruit, rotating as you go. Over a medium bowl, run the paring knife between the segments and the membranes to remove the segments (the bowl will collect excess grapefruit juice, which is used in the dressing). Squeeze juice from any pulp that remains attached to the pith and discard the pith and peel. Place the segments in a large bowl.

2 In the medium bowl with the grapefruit juice, add the lime zest, lime juice, and olive oil and whisk until combined. Season with salt and pepper. Set aside. Add the basil right before serving.

3 **For the Salad:** In the large bowl with the grapefruit segments, add the romaine, radicchio, jicama, avocado, onion, and basil to combine. Drizzle the dressing around the rim of the salad bowl and toss to evenly coat. Sprinkle with pistachios, season with additional salt and pepper, and serve.

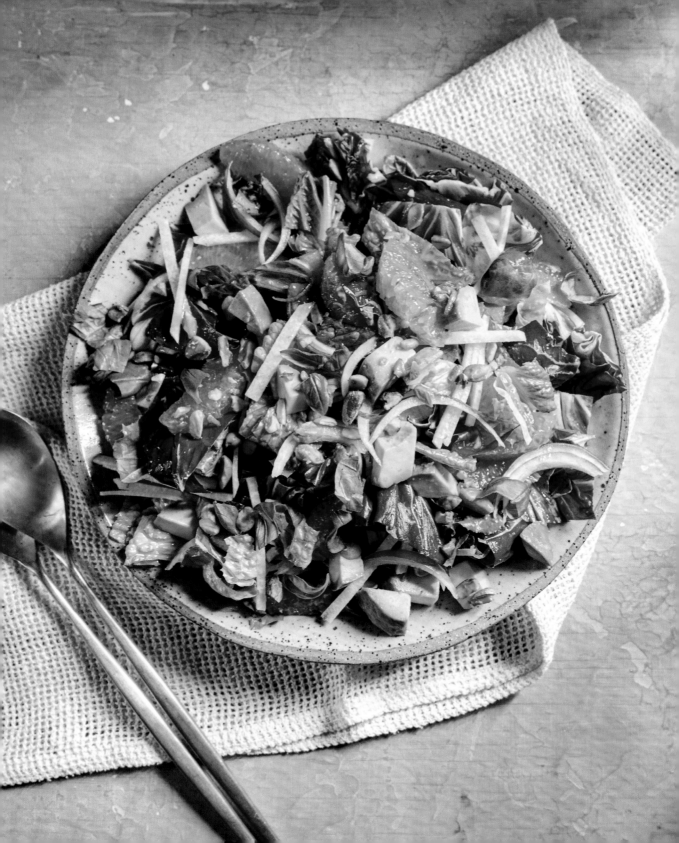

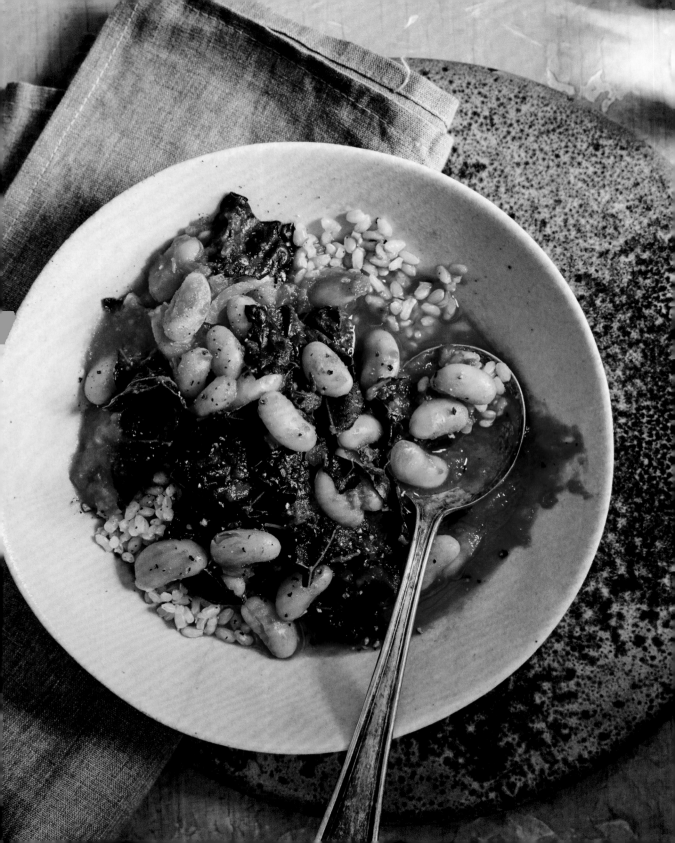

Portuguese Spicy White Bean Stew

with Tomatoes and Kale

PREP TIME// 15 minutes

COOK TIME// 35 minutes

SERVES// 4

2 tablespoons avocado oil

1 small yellow onion, diced

3 garlic cloves, minced

1 tablespoon fresh thyme or
2 teaspoons dried

½ teaspoon red chili flakes

Sea salt and freshly ground black
pepper to taste

1 (28-ounce) can crushed tomatoes

4 cups low-sodium vegetable stock

2 (15-ounce) cans cannellini beans,
drained and rinsed

1 bunch lacinato kale or another green,
stems removed, and chopped

2 cups cooked brown rice, to serve

A stew on a weeknight seems impossible, but this is a quick veggie stew that's full of flavor in under an hour. I was inspired to make a completely plant-based stew similar to caldo verde, a traditional Portuguese soup made with spicy sausage, a green (like kale), and potatoes.

1 In a large Dutch oven or heavy-bottomed pot, heat the avocado oil over medium-high heat. Add the onion and garlic and allow to cook for about 4 minutes, or until softened. Add the thyme, chili flakes, and salt, and pepper, and cook for an additional minute.

2 Add the tomatoes, stock, and cannellini beans. Bring to a boil, then reduce the heat and allow to simmer for 25 to 30 minutes, adding the kale during the last 10 minutes of cooking, until the flavors meld together. Season again with salt and pepper and serve over brown rice.

TIP: This is the perfect cold-weather treat. I like to freeze half this stew to have for an unexpectedly busy week.

Supergreen Pasta

PREP TIME// 10 minutes

COOK TIME// 20 minutes

SERVES// 4

Herby Green Sauce

1 cup packed spinach

3 garlic cloves

½ cup raw walnuts

3 tablespoons fresh flat-leaf parsley

3 tablespoons fresh cilantro

3 tablespoons fresh mint

¼ cup extra-virgin olive oil

2 tablespoons red wine vinegar

2 tablespoons water

½ teaspoon sea salt and freshly
ground black pepper to taste

Pasta

Sea salt to taste

1 (8-ounce) package brown rice penne,
lentil penne, or any plant-based pasta

Head of broccoli (about 1½ pounds),
cut into florets

1 tablespoon avocado oil

Freshly ground black pepper to taste

1 to 2 cups baby spinach (depending
on your desired noodle-to-green ratio)

2 tablespoons roughly chopped fresh
mint, to garnish

2 tablespoons roughly chopped fresh
flat-leaf parsley, to garnish

2 tablespoons roughly chopped fresh
cilantro, to garnish

¼ cup Almond Parmesan (optional;
page 241)

Vegetable-based pastas are an ingredient I always have around because they provide both protein and fiber. The green sauce for this pasta is inspired by classic herb sauces like chimichurri and pesto, using a variety of fresh herbs with a hint of acid from red wine vinegar, plus walnuts for a nutty, creamy texture. It's great not only for pasta but also for roasted veggies, salads, and proteins.

1 **For the Herby Green Sauce:** In the carafe of a high-speed blender, blend the spinach, garlic, walnuts, parsley, cilantro, mint, olive oil, vinegar, and water until well combined. Season with salt and pepper. Set aside.

2 Preheat the oven to 400°F.

3 **For the Pasta:** Bring a large pot of salted water to a boil, add the pasta, and cook for 2 minutes less than the package instructions advise.

4 Meanwhile, line a rimmed baking sheet with parchment paper. On the prepared baking sheet, toss the broccoli with avocado oil and season with salt and pepper. Roast for 15 minutes, tossing halfway through, until golden brown and crisp-tender. When finished roasting, remove the broccoli from the oven and allow to cool slightly.

5 Drain the pasta, lightly rinse, and transfer to a large bowl. Add the green sauce, roasted broccoli, and baby spinach to the bowl with the pasta and toss together. Garnish with the chopped mint, parsley, and cilantro and a sprinkle of "parm" (if using).

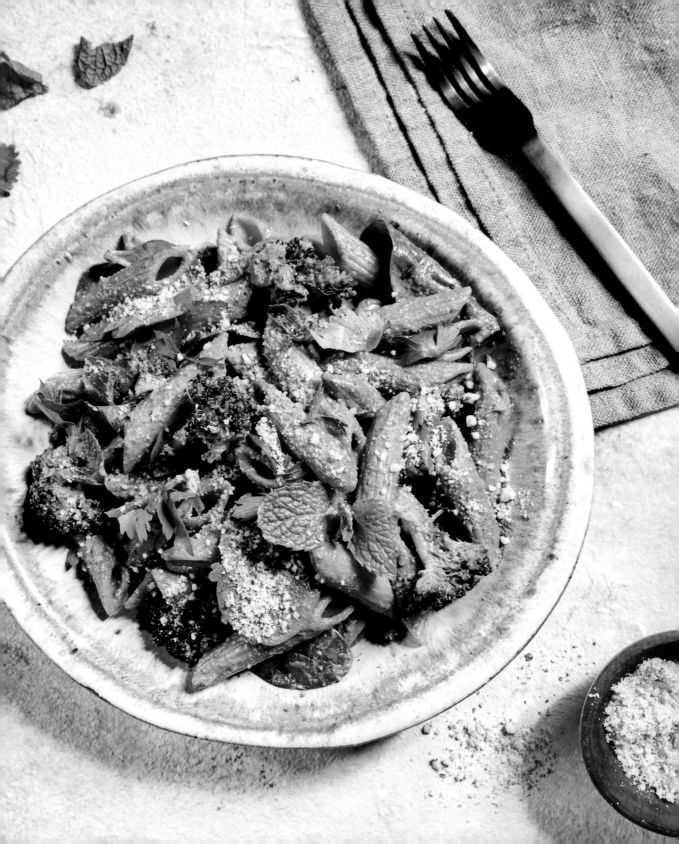

Forbidden Rice Salad

with Roasted Beets and Butternut Squash

PREP TIME// 10 minutes

COOK TIME// 40 minutes

SERVES// 4

Orange Thyme Vinaigrette

2 garlic cloves, minced

1 shallot, chopped

3 tablespoons white wine vinegar

1 navel orange, half zested and all juiced

2 tablespoons fresh thyme or 1 teaspoon dried

⅓ cup extra-virgin olive oil

Sea salt and freshly ground black pepper to taste

Forbidden Rice Salad

1 cup forbidden rice

2 small beets, peeled and cut into ½-inch-thick wedges

¼ cup avocado oil

Sea salt and freshly ground black pepper to taste

14.5 ounces butternut squash, seeded and cut into ½- to ¾-inch cubes (about 3 cups)

3 cups baby arugula

½ cup roasted unsalted pecans, chopped

This salad is ideal to pack for lunch on a workday or even for an adventure. Each bite is full of flavor and texture from the rich forbidden rice to the sweet roasted squash and beets. Forbidden rice has numerous health benefits, too, that shouldn't be ignored. It's high in antioxidants, specifically anthocyanin, which help reduce cardiovascular disease and inflammation and improve brain function.

1 **For the Orange Thyme Vinaigrette:** In a small bowl, whisk together the garlic, shallot, vinegar, orange zest, orange juice, and thyme. While whisking, slowly stream in the olive oil. Season with salt and pepper. Set aside.

2 **For the Forbidden Rice Salad:** Preheat the oven to 400°F. Line two baking sheets with parchment paper.

3 Cook the forbidden rice according to the package instructions.

4 In a medium bowl, toss the beets with 2 tablespoons of the avocado oil and season with salt and pepper. Place on the first prepared baking sheet.

5 Toss the butternut squash with the remaining 2 tablespoons oil and season with salt and pepper. Place on the second prepared baking sheet. Roast the beets and squash for 35 to 40 minutes, until tender, flipping halfway through.

6 Once the rice is cooked, allow to cool slightly, then transfer to a large bowl. Add the beets, squash, arugula, and pecans and toss together. Drizzle half the vinaigrette around the rim of the bowl and toss once again to combine. Add additional dressing to your liking or reserve the remaining for another use. Serve. Salad will keep for up to 3 days.

TIP: This is a great make-ahead salad. Combine all the ingredients, except for the arugula, and allow to marinate in the fridge for up to 1 day. Toss the arugula into the salad right before serving.

Dom Scott's Coconut Curry Rice Bowl

ATHLETE RECIPE: Dominique Scott is a two-time track-and-field Olympian representing her home country of South Africa and Adidas International. Dom was a five-time NCAA Champion for the University of Arkansas Razorbacks. Dom now lives and trains in Boulder, Colorado.

"I love this veggie-packed curry recipe. It's a quick and delicious weeknight meal that's full of flavor and texture. It's also gluten- and dairy-free, making it one of my favorite post-workout dinners since it's easy on the stomach."

1 For the Coconut Rice: In a medium saucepan, combine the white rice, curry paste, coconut milk, water, and salt. Bring to a boil, stirring occasionally. Reduce the heat, cover with a lid, and allow to simmer for 15 minutes, or until the rice is fluffy and cooked through (there will be some extra liquid in the pan that will be absorbed after sitting).

2 Once rice is cooked, remove from the heat, keeping the lid on to steam for 10 additional minutes. Fluff rice with a fork.

3 For the Vegetables: Meanwhile, in a large sauté pan heat the coconut oil over medium heat. Add the onion and allow to cook for 3 to 5 minutes, until softened, stirring occasionally. Add the garlic and cook for an additional minute.

4 Add the carrots, bell pepper, green beans, and chickpeas and cook for 7 to 8 minutes, stirring occasionally, until the vegetables are almost tender but still have some bite. Add the turmeric during the final minute of cooking and season with salt.

5 Add the rice to the sauté pan and stir until combined with the vegetables. Season with additional salt. Garnish with the basil and cashews. Divide among four bowls and serve with lime wedges.

PREP TIME// 15 minutes
COOK TIME// 30 minutes
SERVES// 4

Coconut Rice

1 cup long-grain white rice

2 to 3 tablespoons Thai red curry paste (depending on your spice preference)

1 (13.5-ounce) can light coconut milk, well shaken

½ cup water

1 teaspoon sea salt

Vegetables

1 tablespoon coconut oil

1 small yellow onion, chopped

2 garlic cloves, minced

2 large carrots, thinly sliced into half-moons

1 small red bell pepper, cored, seeded, and thinly sliced

8 ounces green beans, trimmed and cut into 1½-inch pieces

1 (15-ounce) can chickpeas, drained and rinsed

½ teaspoon ground turmeric

Sea salt to taste

¼ cup torn fresh basil, to garnish

½ cup roasted unsalted cashews, roughly chopped, to garnish

Lime wedges, to serve

Kate Courtney's Fish Taco Bowl

ATHLETE RECIPE: Kate Courtney is a professional mountain bike racer for the SCOTT-SRAM MTB Racing Team. Kate is the 2019 Elite XCO World Cup Overall Champion, the 2018 Elite XCO World Champion, and a two-time Elite US National Champion. She grew up in Marin County, California, at the base of Mount Tamalpais, the birthplace of mountain biking. Kate is also a graduate of Stanford University with a bachelor's in human biology.

"I love simple but flavorful dishes that are packed with protein and healthy fats to fuel hard training weeks. I have also always been a big fan of tacos. This is where I got my idea to create a fish taco bowl. By making this bowl with brown rice, I'm able to get in some extra carbs for hard weeks, and the fish, avocado salsa, and black beans help make it a balanced and delicious meal. This recipe is a great way to combine fresh and healthy ingredients that meet my nutritional needs and keep Taco Tuesday fun and tasty!"

1 For the Spiced Fish: Preheat the oven to 425°F. Line a baking sheet with parchment paper.

2 Prepare a dredging station with three shallow bowls. In the first bowl, mix the oat flour and Tajin seasoning. In the second bowl, whisk the eggs. Place the cornmeal in the final bowl. Season each with salt and pepper.

3 Dredge the first piece of fish in the oat flour mixture, shaking off any excess. Dip into the eggs and then the cornmeal, pressing gently to ensure the cornmeal sticks. Place on the prepared baking sheet and repeat with the remaining pieces of fish. Spray the top of the fish with cooking spray and bake for 25 to 28 minutes, until golden brown and fish is cooked through. Remove from the oven and season with additional salt and pepper.

4 For the Avocado Salsa: In a medium bowl, combine the avocado, pineapple, tomato, shallot, jalapeño, garlic, cilantro, and lime juice. Season with salt and pepper and toss to combine. Set aside to marinate.

5 For the Bowl: In a small bowl, whisk together the lime juice and olive oil and season with salt and pepper. In a large bowl, toss the brown rice and cabbage to evenly coat. Divide the mixture among four bowls. Top with black beans, tortilla chips, pumpkin seeds, the salsa, and fish. Serve with hot sauce (if using) and lime wedges.

PREP TIME// 20 minutes
COOK TIME// 15 minutes
SERVES// 4

Spiced Fish

¼ cup oat flour

2 tablespoons Tajin seasoning (or chili lime seasoning)

3 large eggs, lightly beaten

1 cup yellow cornmeal

Sea salt and freshly ground black pepper to taste

1 pound skinless rock cod, cut into 2 × 1-inch pieces

Extra-virgin olive oil cooking spray, for greasing

Avocado Salsa

1 avocado, peeled, pitted, and diced

1 cup chopped pineapple

1 large tomato, seeded and diced

1 small shallot, chopped

1 jalapeño, seeded and chopped

1 garlic clove, grated

⅓ cup chopped fresh cilantro

1 to 2 limes, juiced

Sea salt and freshly ground black pepper to taste

Bowl

¼ cup fresh lime juice

¼ cup extra-virgin olive oil

Sea salt and freshly ground black pepper to taste

2 cups cooked brown rice, warmed

2 cups thinly sliced red cabbage

1 (15-ounce) can black beans, drained and rinsed

1 cup baked corn tortilla chips, crushed

¼ cup roasted and salted pumpkin seeds

Hot sauce (optional), to serve

Lime wedges, to serve

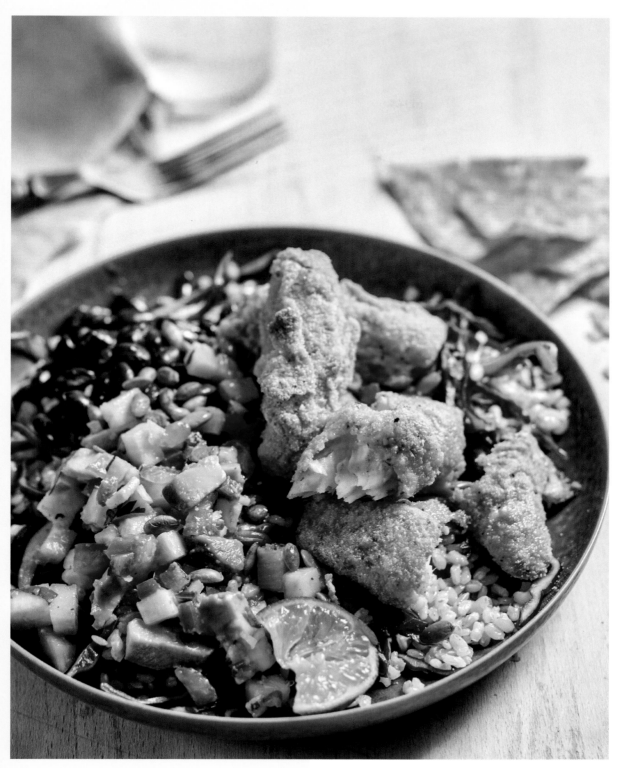

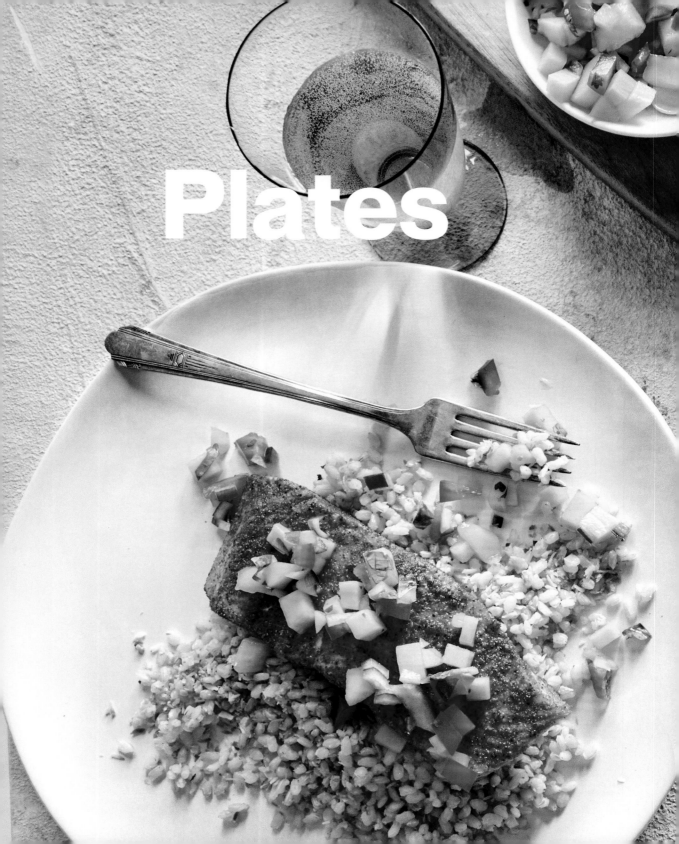

Plates

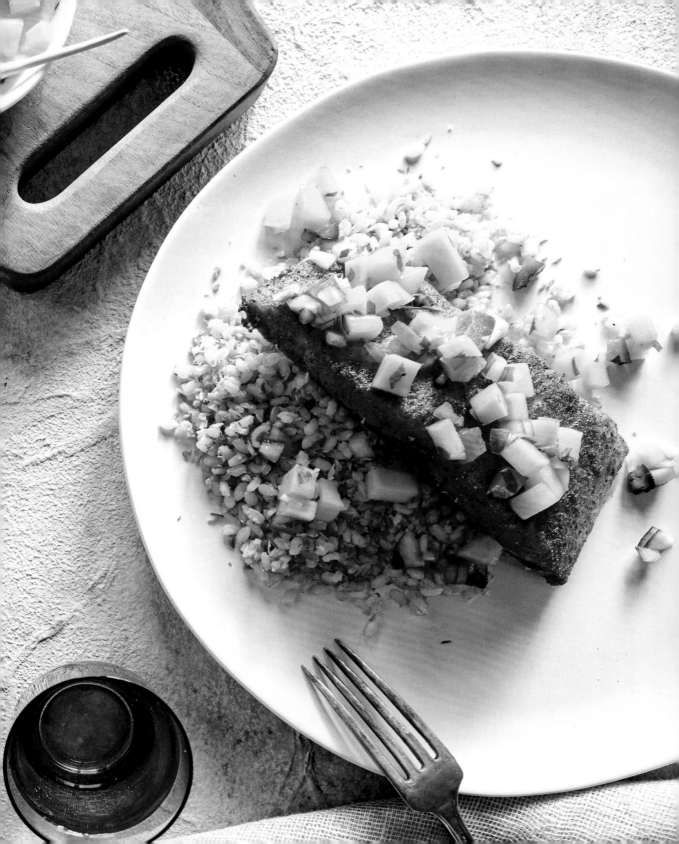

These are what I call the showstoppers of the book! These recipes really aren't intimidating: I promise they are both easy to prepare and full of great flavor. When thinking about the recipes I wanted to include and develop for this chapter, I loved the idea of putting flavor twists on classic recipes that I've always loved by incorporating spices, veggies, and whole grains. Salmon burgers have always been my go-to summer recipe, and with my Ginger Pineapple Salmon Burger (page 122), I decided to add some Asian flavors as well as pineapple for a fresh bite. For my Tempeh and Brussels Sprouts Tacos with Pickled Cabbage (page 124), I wanted to use the nuttiness and rich protein of tempeh in combination with fiber-rich Brussels sprouts and a Mexican spice blend for a plant-based taco unlike any other. A lot of these recipes also use vegetables and whole grains in unique ways that you've probably never thought of or tried, like using butternut squash as the sauce base for the Butternut Squash Mac and Cheese (page 127) and quinoa as the crust in the Quinoa Crust Pizza with Broccoli Rabe and Almond Ricotta (page 135). Use these recipes to your meal-prep and entertaining advantage during the week—they are definitely crowd-pleasers!

Ginger Pineapple Salmon Burger

PREP TIME// 15 minutes +
30 minutes refrigeration

COOK TIME// 35 minutes

SERVES// 6

Salmon Burger

⅓ cup roughly chopped fresh cilantro

¼ cup roughly chopped scallions
(white and light green parts)

3 garlic cloves

1 (1-inch) piece of ginger, peeled and
roughly chopped

2 tablespoons Dijon mustard

2 tablespoons apricot jam

1 teaspoon hot sauce

½ teaspoon chili powder

1 teaspoon miso paste

1 pound skinless salmon fillet, cut into
1-inch pieces

½ cup ground flaxseed

½ cup fresh pineapple, diced small

½ cup cooked short-grain brown rice,
cooled

Sea salt to taste

Avocado oil cooking spray

Salad

2 tablespoons avocado oil

4 pineapple spears

1 (5-ounce) package mixed greens

1 avocado, pitted, peeled, and mashed

Sesame Miso Sauce

2 tablespoons white miso paste

1 tablespoon toasted sesame oil

1 lime, zested and juiced

¼ cup warm water

This burger is one of my meal-prep recipe staples. I make the full recipe and freeze some of the raw salmon patties for another easy weeknight dinner. This recipe is packed full of flavor with tang from the ginger, mustard, and miso paste, and sweetness from the apricot jam and pineapple. The hot sauce and chili powder also give the salmon a slight kick, highlighting all the different flavors in a burger that everyone loves.

1 **For the Salmon Burgers:** Line a baking sheet with parchment paper.

2 In the bowl of a food processor fitted with the blade attachment, pulse the cilantro, scallions, garlic, ginger, mustard, apricot jam, hot sauce, chili powder, and miso paste until finely chopped, almost like a paste. Add the salmon and pulse until roughly chopped (be sure the salmon isn't too finely ground).

3 Transfer the salmon mixture to a large bowl and gently fold in the flaxseed, pineapple, and brown rice. Season with salt. Form into six ½-cup patties. Place on the prepared baking sheet, cover loosely with plastic wrap, and refrigerate for 30 minutes.

4 Preheat the oven to 425°F.

5 Remove the patties from the refrigerator and spray the tops with avocado oil. Bake for 20 to 25 minutes, flipping halfway through, until golden brown, opaque, and cooked through.

6 **For the Salad:** In a large cast-iron skillet or nonstick sauté pan, heat 1 tablespoon of the avocado oil over medium-high heat. Brush the pineapple spears with the remaining 1 tablespoon oil and place in the pan to cook for 3 minutes per side, or until lightly charred. Remove and chop into smaller pieces.

7 **For the Sesame Miso Sauce:** In a small bowl, whisk together the miso paste, sesame oil, lime zest, lime juice, and warm water until smooth.

8 To assemble, divide the mixed greens among four plates and top with the chopped charred pineapple. Add a salmon burger and top the burger with avocado mash and a pinch of salt. Drizzle with sauce and serve immediately.

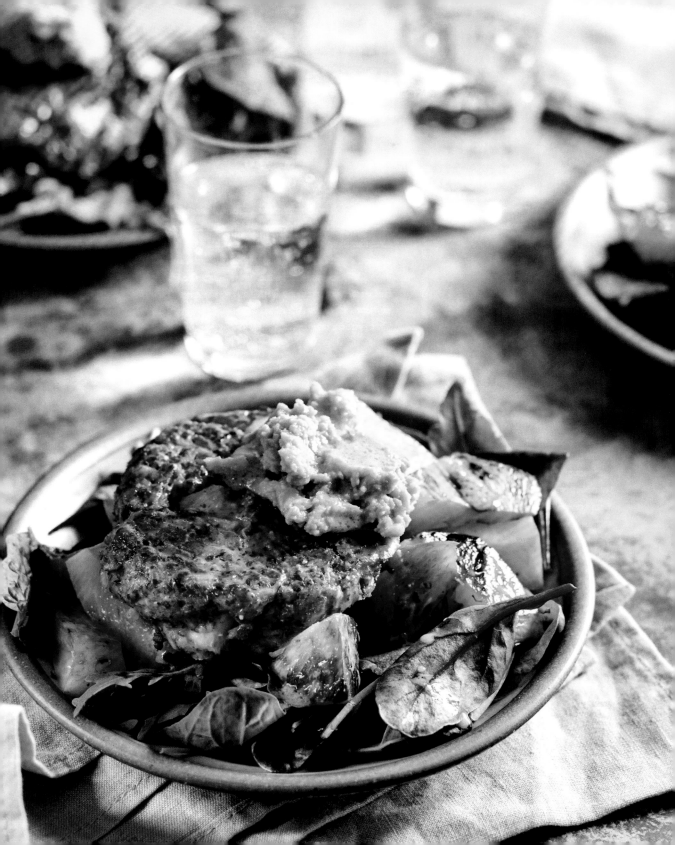

Tempeh and Brussels Sprouts Tacos

with Pickled Cabbage

PREP TIME// 30 minutes

COOK TIME// 35 minutes

SERVES// 4

Pickled Cabbage

2 cups shredded red cabbage

1 teaspoon cumin seed, cracked

1 cup rice wine vinegar

½ cup water

2 teaspoons sea salt

Spiced Tempeh and Brussels Sprouts

Sea salt to taste

1 (8-ounce) package tempeh, cut into ½-inch pieces

1 tablespoon chili powder

1 teaspoon ground cumin

¼ teaspoon cayenne pepper

1 (10-ounce) container Brussels sprouts, trimmed and halved

2 tablespoons avocado oil

Tacos

8 (8-inch) brown rice tortillas

½ cup store-bought salsa verde

1 avocado, pitted, peeled, and thinly sliced

¼ cup fresh cilantro leaves

2 limes, cut into wedges, to serve

How to prepare tempeh is one of the questions I get asked the most. I like to say tempeh is tofu's healthier cousin since it's less processed. It comes in an almost cake-like block that is fairly dense with an earthy, nutty flavor. It's made from cooked soybeans that go through a fermentation process so they are easier to digest. Whole grains and other flavorings can be added to tempeh as well. I always boil or steam my tempeh for 10 minutes before cooking to further tenderize the soybeans for easier digestion. Tempeh also has several health benefits: it's high in fiber, protein, magnesium, B vitamins, and probiotics from fermentation.

1 **For the Pickled Cabbage:** Place the cabbage and cumin seed in a large heatproof bowl or jar. In a small saucepan, bring the vinegar, water, and salt to a simmer until the salt dissolves, about 3 minutes.

2 Pour the brine over the cabbage and allow to sit at room temperature to soften and cool until ready to serve.

3 **For the Spiced Tempeh and Brussels Sprouts:** Preheat the oven to 400°F. Line a baking sheet with parchment paper.

4 Bring a large pot of salted water to a boil. Add the tempeh and allow to boil for 10 minutes, or until softened. Drain and pat very dry.

5 In a small bowl, mix together the chili powder, cumin, and cayenne. Toss the tempeh and Brussels sprouts together on the prepared baking sheet. Sprinkle with spice mixture and drizzle with avocado oil. Toss everything again to make sure it's evenly coated, and season with salt. Roast for 25 to 30 minutes, flipping halfway through, until the tempeh is golden brown and Brussels sprouts are tender.

6 **For the Tacos:** Over a low open gas flame or in a large cast-iron skillet, carefully place the tortilla on top of the flame or in the skillet and allow it to warm and lightly char.

7 To assemble, place some of the tempeh and Brussels sprouts in each tortilla and top with salsa verde, pickled cabbage, avocado, and cilantro leaves. Serve with lime wedges.

TIP: This taco is also great using your protein of choice. Toss the protein in the spices and sear or roast until cooked through.

Homemade BBQ Salmon

PREP TIME// 10 minutes

COOK TIME// 14 minutes

SERVES// 4

BBQ Sauce

¼ cup fruit-sweetened apricot jam

3 tablespoons liquid aminos (I like Bragg)

3 tablespoons Dijon mustard

3 tablespoons sriracha

3 tablespoons fresh lemon juice

2 tablespoons apple cider vinegar

1½ teaspoons onion powder

1½ teaspoons garlic powder

½ teaspoon smoked paprika

1 tablespoon tomato paste

Sea salt to taste

Salmon

4 (4- to 6-ounce) skin-on salmon fillets

2 scallions (white and light green parts), thinly sliced, to garnish

¼ cup chopped fresh cilantro, to garnish

Homemade BBQ sauce was one of the first recipes I made when I started to cook. The secret ingredient in the sauce is fruit-sweetened apricot jam. It adds the perfect touch of natural sweetness without any added sugars. I use this sauce on fish as well as tofu and love to serve with Vegan Mexican Street Corn (page 150) on the side.

1 **For the BBQ Sauce:** In a small bowl, whisk together the jam, liquid aminos, mustard, sriracha, lemon juice, vinegar, onion powder, garlic powder, paprika, and tomato paste. Season with salt and set aside until ready to use.

2 **For the Salmon:** Preheat the oven to 425°F.

3 Line a baking sheet with parchment paper. Place the salmon fillets on the prepared baking sheet and spoon over the BBQ sauce. Bake for 12 to 14 minutes, until pink and opaque, the sauce is caramelized, and the fish flakes easily with a fork. Divide among four plates, garnish with scallions and cilantro, and serve.

TIP: Also try this with tofu! Be sure to press the tofu (see step 1 page 45) and pat very dry before cutting into 1-inch squares, tossing with BBQ sauce, and baking for 15 to 20 minutes, until lightly golden.

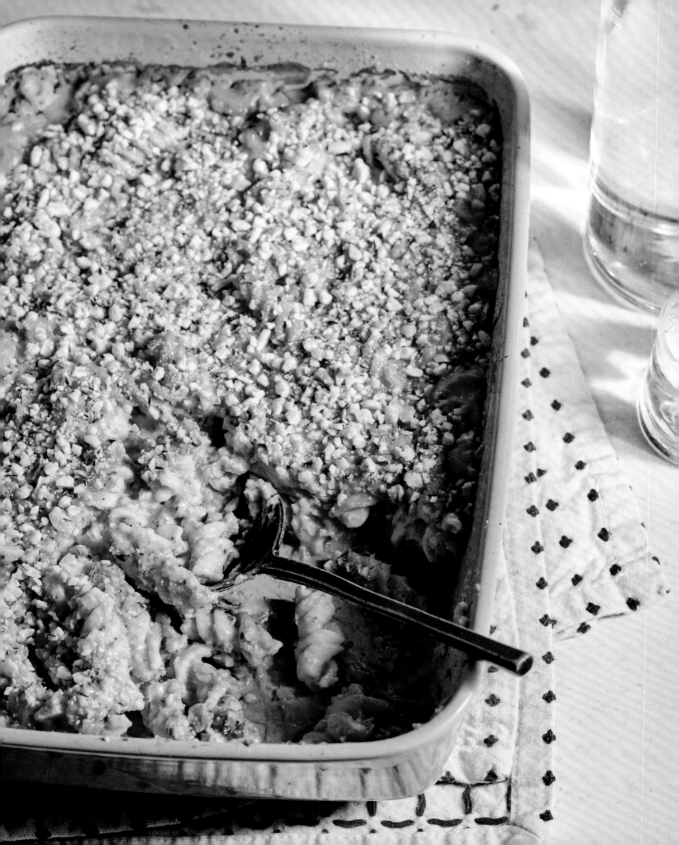

Butternut Squash Mac and Cheese

PREP TIME// 15 minutes
COOK TIME// 38 minutes
SERVES// 4 to 6

Topping

½ cup raw cashews

2 tablespoons hemp seeds

2 tablespoons nutritional yeast

1 teaspoon garlic powder

½ teaspoon onion powder

½ teaspoon dried thyme

Sea salt to taste

Mac and Cheese

Sea salt to taste

1 pound brown rice or chickpea rotini

3 tablespoons avocado oil

1 medium yellow onion, diced

2 garlic cloves, sliced

1 teaspoon dried thyme

14.5 ounces butternut squash, peeled, seeded, and cubed (about 3 cups)

2 cups low-sodium vegetable stock

½ cup unsweetened nut milk

¼ cup nutritional yeast

Freshly ground black pepper to taste

Pureed butternut squash is the key ingredient to transforming this sauce into a veggie-forward recipe. This sauce is rich in vitamins A and C, which help eye, bone, and immune system health, and it is also a great source of manganese, which helps with building bone tissue. The nutty topping on this dish is my favorite part since it adds extra cheesy flavor as well as a crunch from the cashews and hemp seeds.

1 **For the Topping:** In the bowl of a food processor fitted with the blade attachment, pulse the cashews, hemp seeds, nutritional yeast, garlic powder, onion powder, and thyme until roughly chopped to resemble coarse bread crumbs. Season with salt and set aside.

2 **For the Mac and Cheese:** Bring a large pot of salted water to a boil, add the pasta, and cook for 2 minutes less than the package instructions advise. Drain and rinse under cold water. Place in a large bowl and set aside.

3 In a heavy-bottomed pot or Dutch oven, heat 2 tablespoons of the avocado oil over medium-high heat. Add the onion and cook for about 4 minutes, or until softened. Add the garlic and thyme and season with salt and cook for an additional minute.

4 Add the squash and stock to the pot and season again with salt. Bring to a boil, then reduce the heat and allow to simmer for 20 minutes, or until the squash is very tender.

5 Preheat the oven to 400°F.

6 Carefully transfer the squash mixture to the carafe of a high-speed blender. Add the nut milk and nutritional yeast and blend until smooth. Season with salt and pepper to taste.

7 Pour the sauce over the pasta and mix to evenly coat. Transfer to an 11 × 7-inch baking dish. Sprinkle the topping over the pasta and drizzle with remaining 1 tablespoon avocado oil. Bake for 10 to 12 minutes, until bubbling and golden. Allow to cool for 5 minutes before serving.

Miso-Glazed Eggplant

with Spiced Farro

PREP TIME// 20 minutes

COOK TIME// 35 minutes

SERVES// 4

Miso-Glazed Eggplant

4 medium eggplants, halved lengthwise

2 tablespoons avocado oil

Sea salt to taste

¼ cup yellow or white miso paste

2 tablespoons rice wine vinegar

2 tablespoons water

Spiced Farro

½ cup farro

2 tablespoons avocado oil

1 small yellow onion, diced

2 garlic cloves, minced

1 teaspoon ground turmeric

1 teaspoon ground coriander

½ teaspoon ground cumin

½ teaspoon ground cinnamon

Sea salt and freshly ground black pepper to taste

6 tablespoons fresh lemon juice

⅓ cup pitted Medjool dates, chopped

3 tablespoons chopped fresh mint

3 tablespoons chopped fresh flat-leaf parsley

3 tablespoons tahini

⅓ cup pomegranate seeds, to garnish

Eggplant happens to be one of my ideal vegetables for roasting. The eggplant caramelizes in the oven and becomes tender and soft. The miso sauce adds a salty flavor that browns beautifully underneath the broiler. To finish, I love topping roasted eggplant with a fresh salad or herby whole grain, and this spiced farro does just the trick. It has both warm spices as well as mint and parsley, giving this recipe so many levels of flavor.

1 **For the Miso-Glazed Eggplant:** Place one oven rack in the lower third of the oven and a second rack underneath the broiler. Preheat the oven to 425°F.

2 Line a baking sheet with parchment paper. Using a paring knife, cut a crisscross diamond pattern into the flesh of the eggplant, scoring the surface. Brush both sides of the eggplants with avocado oil and season with salt. Place on the prepared baking sheet and roast on the lower oven rack for 25 to 30 minutes, until tender.

3 Meanwhile, in a small bowl, whisk together the miso paste, vinegar, and water until smooth. Once the eggplant is tender, remove from the oven and preheat the broiler. Spoon the miso mixture over the eggplant and return to the top rack of the oven underneath the broiler. Allow to broil 2 to 6 minutes, until deep golden brown. (Keep an eye on the miso sauce so it doesn't burn!)

4 **For the Spiced Farro:** Cook the farro according to the package instructions.

5 Meanwhile, in a large sauté pan, heat the avocado oil over medium-high heat. Add the onion and garlic and cook for 5 to 6 minutes, until lightly browned. Add the turmeric, coriander, cumin, and cinnamon and allow the spices to toast an additional minute. Season with salt and pepper.

6 Add the farro, season again with salt and pepper, and stir to combine. Allow to cook for another 2 to 3 minutes, until fragrant.

7 Remove from the heat and allow to cool for 5 minutes. Stir in half the lemon juice, the dates, mint, and parsley.

8 In a small bowl, whisk together the remaining lemon juice and the tahini.

9 Place the eggplant halves on a serving dish and spoon the warm farro on top. Scatter the pomegranate seeds over the top, finish with a drizzle of lemon tahini sauce, and serve.

TIP: If you aren't a fan of eggplant, this miso glaze can be used on all different vegetables. It adds a delicious salty, umami flavor.

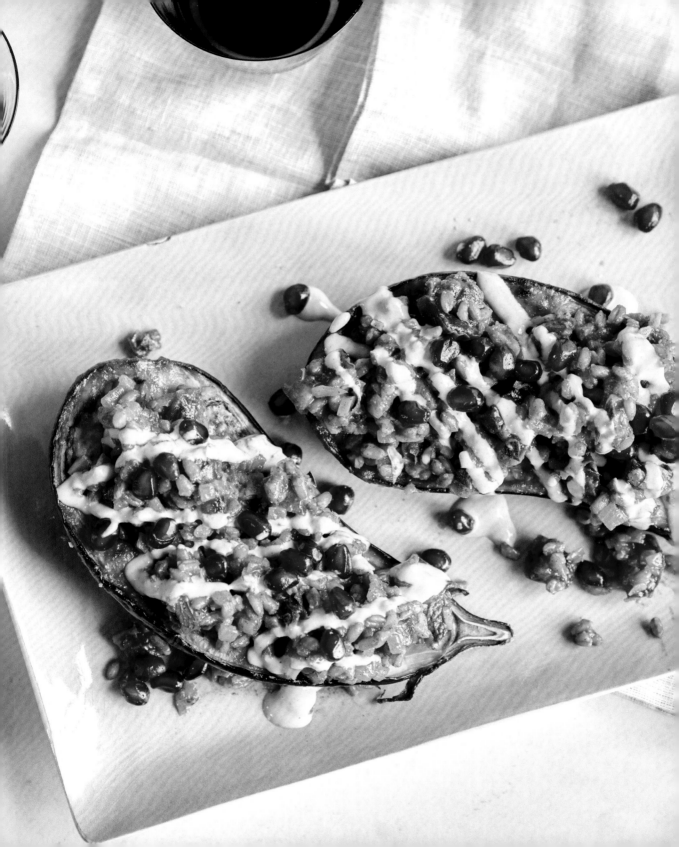

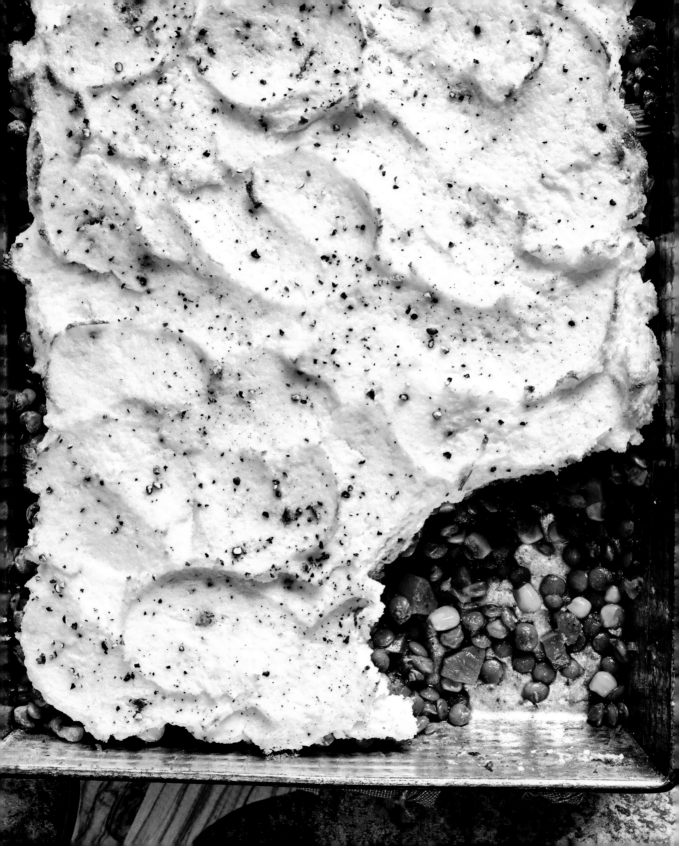

Veggie Shepherd's Pie

with Cauliflower Mash

PREP TIME // 20 minutes

COOK TIME // 1 hour

SERVES // 4 to 6

Cauliflower Topping

Sea salt to taste

Medium head of cauliflower
(about 3 pounds), cut into florets
(about 7 cups)

3 tablespoons avocado oil

Freshly ground black pepper to taste

Lentil Filling

2 tablespoons avocado oil, plus
additional to drizzle

1 small yellow onion, diced

2 carrots, diced small

2 ribs celery, diced small

2 garlic cloves, minced

1 teaspoon dried thyme

1 teaspoon dried rosemary

2 tablespoons tomato paste

1½ cups French green lentils, rinsed
and picked over for stones

Sea salt and freshly ground black
pepper to taste

4 cups water

1 cup fresh or frozen corn kernels,
thawed if frozen

1 cup frozen peas, thawed

This shepherd's pie recipe is my kitchen staples dinner since I usually have all the ingredients already stocked in my pantry and fridge. The savory iron-rich lentils, seasoned with dried thyme and rosemary, consist of more than 25 percent protein, making them a flavorful, hearty filling. For the topping, cauliflower mash is a fun swap for the classic mashed russet potato. This is a great crowd-pleaser, especially in the colder months, and you can use whatever seasonal root vegetables you have on hand.

1 **For the Cauliflower Topping:** Bring a large pot of salted water to a boil. Add the cauliflower florets and allow to boil for 6 to 8 minutes, until very tender. Reserve ¼ cup of the cooking water. Drain the cauliflower.

2 Transfer the tender cauliflower florets and reserved cooking liquid to the bowl of a food processor fitted with the blade attachment and add the avocado oil. Blend until very smooth. Season with salt and pepper and set aside.

3 **For the Lentil Filling:** Preheat the oven to 400°F.

4 In a large heavy-bottomed pot, heat the avocado oil over medium-high heat. Add the onion, carrots, and celery and cook for about 5 minutes, or until softened and lightly golden. Add the garlic, thyme, rosemary, tomato paste, and lentils and cook another minute. Season with salt and pepper and add the water. Bring to a boil, then reduce the heat and allow to simmer for 25 to 30 minutes; stir occasionally, until lentils are just tender.

5 Stir in the corn and peas and season with salt and pepper. Remove from the heat and pour the lentils into an 11 × 7-inch baking dish. Spread the cauliflower over the top of the lentils. Drizzle with additional avocado oil.

6 Place the baking dish in the oven for 10 to 12 minutes, until warmed through. Allow to cool for 10 minutes before serving.

Pomegranate Pecan-Crusted Halibut

with Brussels Sprouts and Lentils

PREP TIME// 15 minutes +
10 minutes soaking
COOK TIME// 25 minutes
SERVES// 4

Pomegranate Pecan-Crusted Fish

Avocado oil cooking spray, for greasing (I use a Misto)

½ cup pitted Medjool dates, halved

½ cup warm pomegranate juice

4 (4- to 6-ounce) halibut fillets or fish of choice

1 tablespoon avocado oil

Sea salt to taste

1 cup raw pecans, chopped

Brussels Sprouts and Lentils

¾ cup French green lentils, rinsed and picked through for stones

6 cups shredded Brussels sprouts

2 tablespoons avocado oil

Sea salt and freshly ground black pepper to taste

¼ cup fresh lemon juice

¼ cup extra-virgin olive oil

½ cup roasted and salted pumpkin seeds

½ cup golden raisins

I love the crunch and deep rich flavor that nuts add to a perfectly cooked fillet. Here, we are also making a simple pomegranate glaze that adds a sweet and tangy finish to the recipe as well as contributes some amazing health benefits. Pomegranate juice is actually three times higher in antioxidants than green tea. These antioxidants help reduce inflammation and cell damage.

1 **For the Pomegranate Pecan-Crusted Fish:** Preheat the oven to 425°F. Line a baking sheet with parchment paper and grease with cooking spray.

2 In a small bowl, combine the dates and warm pomegranate juice and allow to sit for 10 minutes, or until the dates have softened. Transfer the mixture to the bowl of a food processor fitted with the blade attachment and blend until smooth. Return to the same small bowl and set aside.

3 Place the halibut fillets on the prepared baking sheet and brush the tops with the avocado oil. Spoon the pomegranate glaze over the fillets and season with salt. Press ¼ cup of the chopped pecans onto the top of each fillet.

4 Roast the halibut on the top rack of the oven for 12 to 15 minutes, until opaque, cooked through, and flakes easily with a fork.

5 **For the Brussels Sprouts and Lentils:** Cook the lentils according to the package instructions.

6 While the lentils are cooking, line a second baking sheet with parchment paper. On the prepared baking sheet, toss the Brussels sprouts with the avocado oil and season with salt and pepper. Roast the Brussels sprouts on the bottom rack of the oven for 12 to 14 minutes, tossing halfway through, until golden brown. Allow to cool for 5 minutes.

7 Meanwhile, in a small bowl, whisk together the lemon juice and olive oil. Season with salt and pepper. Drain the lentils and toss together with the Brussels sprouts, pumpkin seeds, golden raisins, and lemon dressing. Divide among four bowls and top with a piece of halibut.

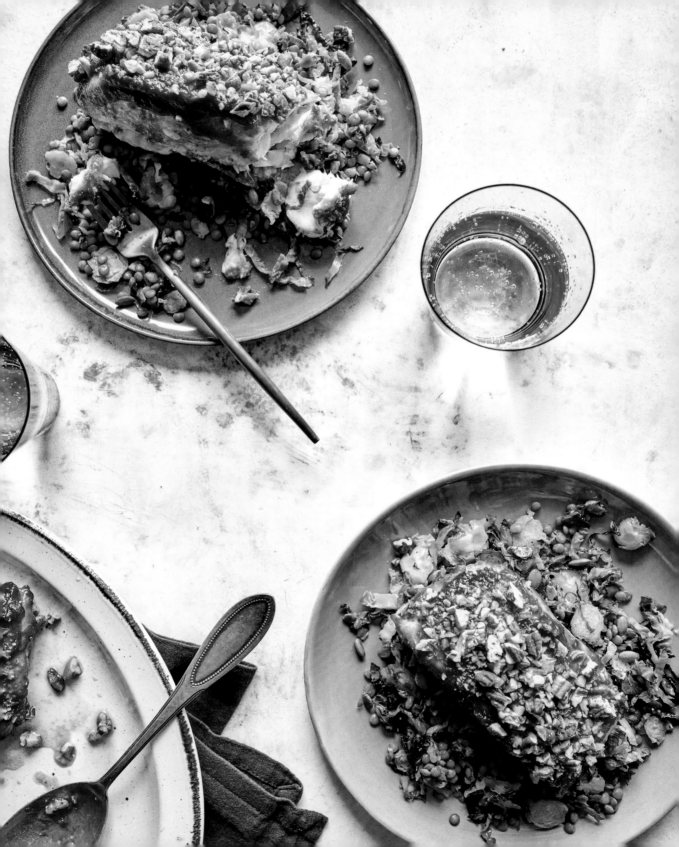

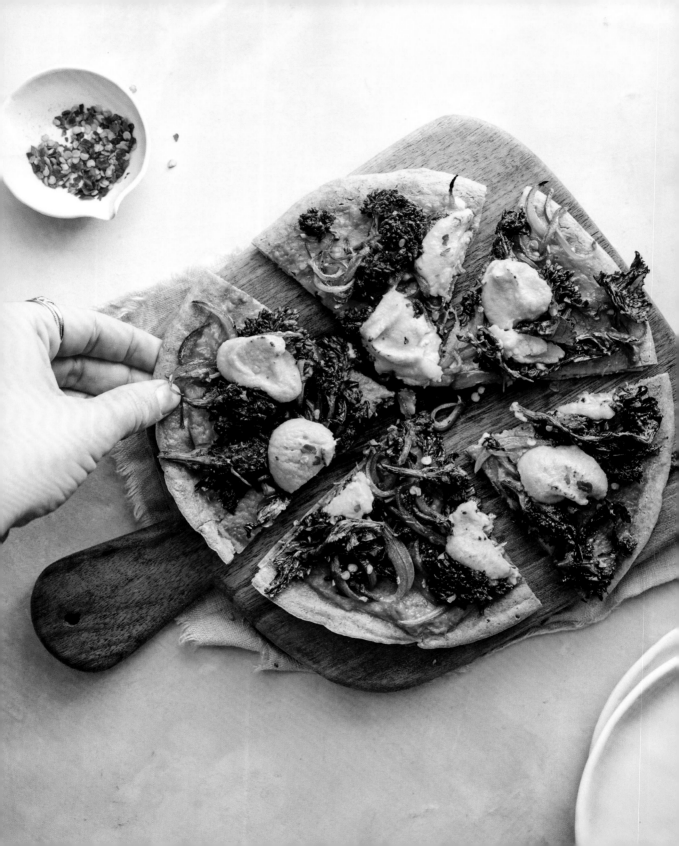

Quinoa Crust Pizza

with Broccoli Rabe and Almond Ricotta

PREP TIME// 20 minutes + soaking for 5 hours or overnight

COOK TIME// 30 minutes

SERVES// 4

Quinoa Crust

1 cup uncooked quinoa (soaked in water to cover for 5 hours or overnight)

1 tablespoon coconut oil

1 teaspoon garlic powder

½ teaspoon baking powder

½ teaspoon sea salt

⅓ cup water

Avocado oil cooking spray, for greasing (I use a Misto)

Pizza

2 tablespoons avocado oil

½ pound broccoli rabe, cut into 1-inch pieces (about 2 packed cups)

1 medium red onion, thinly sliced

2 garlic cloves, minced

Sea salt and freshly ground black pepper to taste

Pinch of red chili flakes (optional)

⅓ cup Roasted Tomato Sauce (page 236), warmed

1 recipe Almond Ricotta (page 242)

If you're looking for an easy, delicious gluten-free pizza crust, look no further—this crust is for you! Blending the soaked, raw quinoa makes a creamy batter that bakes beautifully into a golden crust with crispy edges, perfect for any toppings. Always keep quinoa in your pantry and remember to soak the quinoa for 5 hours before baking for an easy pizza night any day of the week.

1 **For the Quinoa Crust:** Preheat the oven to 400°F.

2 Cut a piece of parchment paper to fit the size of the stainless pizza pan or baking sheet you'll be using. Place the pizza pan without the parchment in the oven to preheat.

3 Drain the soaked quinoa and rinse well in a fine-mesh strainer until the water runs clear. Transfer the quinoa to the carafe of a high-speed blender and add the coconut oil, garlic powder, baking powder, salt, and water. Blend until smooth, almost like the consistency of pancake batter.

4 Grease the parchment paper with cooking spray. Carefully remove the hot pizza pan from the oven, place the parchment paper on top, and spread out the batter to form a 10½-inch pizza round. Bake the crust on the bottom rack of the oven for 22 to 24 minutes, flipping over halfway, until golden brown with crispy edges.

5 **For the Pizza:** Line a second baking sheet with parchment paper. On the prepared baking sheet, toss the avocado oil, broccoli rabe, onion, and garlic until lightly coated. Season with salt and pepper.

6 Roast on the top rack for 20 to 25 minutes, stirring halfway through, until broccoli rabe and onion are lightly browned. Remove from the oven and sprinkle the broccoli rabe with chili flakes, if desired.

7 Preheat the broiler and discard the parchment paper.

8 Spread the tomato sauce on top of the pizza crust. Top with the roasted vegetables and dollops of almond ricotta. Place underneath the broiler for 2 to 5 minutes, until lightly golden and warmed through. Cut the crust into 4 equal slices and serve.

TIPS: If you want to add a flavor to your crust, incorporate chopped fresh herbs and greens, such as parsley, chives, thyme, and spinach.

I like to make a couple of these crusts at a time since they are so quick and easy. I then wrap the cooled crusts in plastic wrap and store in the freezer for a fast pizza meal. Crusts can keep tightly wrapped in the freezer for up to a month.

Sheet Pan Cauliflower and Sweet Potato Curry

PREP TIME// 15 minutes

COOK TIME// 30 minutes

SERVES// 4

¼ cup avocado oil

1 tablespoon curry powder

1 teaspoon ground turmeric

½ teaspoon ground coriander

½ teaspoon cumin seed

Pinch of cayenne pepper

½ large head of cauliflower
(about 2 pounds), cut into small florets
(about 6 cups)

1 (15-ounce) can chickpeas, drained,
rinsed, and patted very dry

2 medium sweet potatoes
(about 2 pounds), peeled and cut
into 1-inch pieces

1 medium red onion, diced large

Sea salt and freshly ground black
pepper to taste

¼ cup chopped fresh cilantro

⅓ cup golden raisins

1 cup plain coconut yogurt, to serve

2 limes, cut into wedges, to serve

Sheet pan recipes are always at the top of my quick-meals list. I like to use whatever veggies I have around plus delicious spices and herbs to add a lot of flavor. Here, the cauliflower and sweet potato are nutrient dense as well as very filling, and the chickpeas add protein for a well-balanced meal. The raisins and yogurt are two surprise additions: the raisins add sweetness while the yogurt adds a tang that rounds out the deep warm curry spices so well.

1 Preheat the oven to 400°F. Line two baking sheets with parchment paper.

2 In a small bowl, whisk together the avocado oil, curry powder, turmeric, coriander, cumin seed, and cayenne. In a large bowl, combine the cauliflower, chickpeas, sweet potatoes, and onion. Drizzle with the avocado oil mixture and toss until evenly coated.

3 Spread evenly onto the prepared baking sheets, being careful not to overcrowd the pans, and season with salt and pepper. Bake for 25 to 30 minutes, stirring halfway through, until golden brown and the sweet potato is tender.

4 Remove from the oven and sprinkle with the cilantro and raisins. Serve with a dollop of yogurt and lime wedges.

TIP: I like to serve this over brown rice or another whole grain for a bowl option.

Vegan Asian Meat Loaf

with Lentils and Shiitakes

PREP TIME// 25 minutes

COOK TIME// 45 minutes

SERVES// 4 to 6

Tomato Glaze

2 tablespoons fruit-sweetened apricot jam

1 tablespoon liquid aminos (I like Bragg)

1 tablespoon tomato paste

1 teaspoon ground flaxseed

¼ cup water

Meat Loaf

Avocado oil cooking spray (I use a Misto)

8 ounces shiitake mushrooms, stems removed, and chopped

2 medium carrots, roughly chopped (about 1 cup)

½ bunch of scallions (white and light green parts), minced

3 garlic cloves, minced

1 (2-inch) piece of ginger, peeled and roughly chopped

2 tablespoons toasted sesame oil

½ cup raw walnuts

½ cup old-fashioned rolled oats

3 cups cooked brown lentils, cooled

1 (8-ounce) can water chestnuts, drained

2 tablespoons ground flaxseed

½ cup fresh flat-leaf parsley

½ teaspoon sea salt

2 tablespoons liquid aminos (I like Bragg)

1 recipe Miso-Mashed Sweet Potatoes with Ginger Shiitakes, to serve (page 153)

This recipe is a new find for me, and I absolutely love all the flavors and textures. I gave this vegetable-based meat loaf an Asian theme because I love shiitake mushrooms as well as the sesame oil, garlic, ginger, and scallion flavors. Be sure to pair this with the Miso-Mashed Sweet Potatoes with Ginger Shiitakes (page 153) for a complete meal.

1 **For the Tomato Glaze:** In a small saucepan, whisk together the apricot jam, liquid aminos, tomato paste, flaxseed, and water. Place over low heat, whisking occasionally, for 3 to 5 minutes, until thickened. Remove from the heat and cover to keep warm.

2 **For the Meat Loaf:** Preheat the oven to 375°F. Grease a 9 × 5-inch loaf pan with cooking spray.

3 In the bowl of a food processor fitted with the blade attachment, pulse the mushrooms, carrots, scallions, garlic, and ginger until finely chopped. In a large sauté pan, heat the sesame oil over medium-high heat. Add the chopped veggie mixture to the pan and allow to cook for 5 to 6 minutes, until softened. Set aside to cool for 5 minutes.

4 Wipe out the food processor, then pulse the walnuts and oats until roughly chopped. Add 1½ cups of the lentils, the water chestnuts, flaxseed, parsley, and salt and pulse until broken up but not smooth (still a little chunky). Remove to a large bowl, add the cooled vegetable mixture, remaining 1½ cups lentils, and liquid aminos. Mix to combine.

5 Scrape the mixture into the loaf pan and smooth the top. Cover with foil and bake for 20 to 25 minutes, until fragrant and browned on top.

6 Remove the meat loaf from the oven, carefully take off the foil, and brush the tomato glaze evenly over the top. Return to the oven, uncovered, and bake for another 10 to 12 minutes, until the sauce is darkened and caramelized. Allow the meat loaf to cool for 10 minutes before slicing. Serve alongside the mashed sweet potatoes.

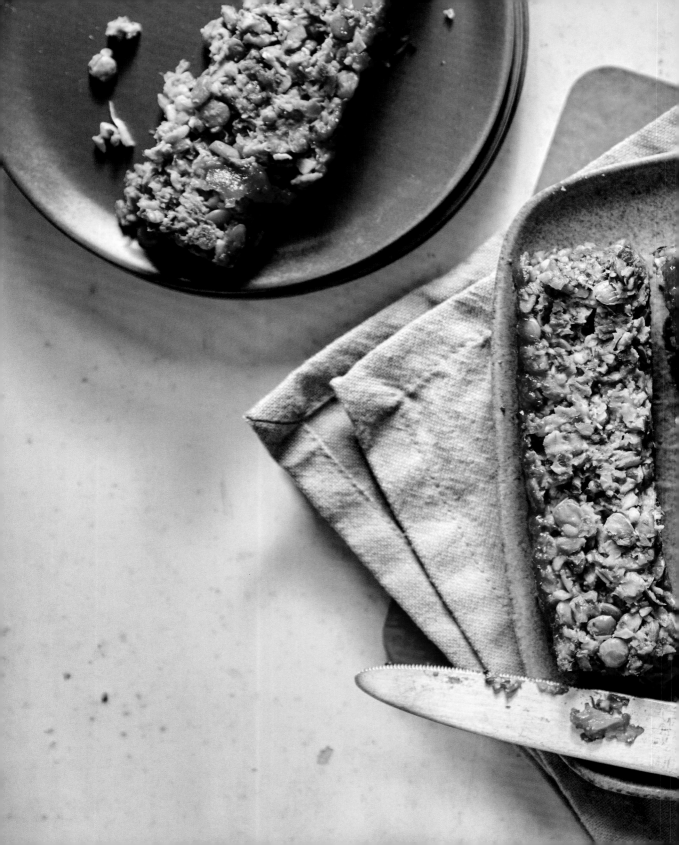

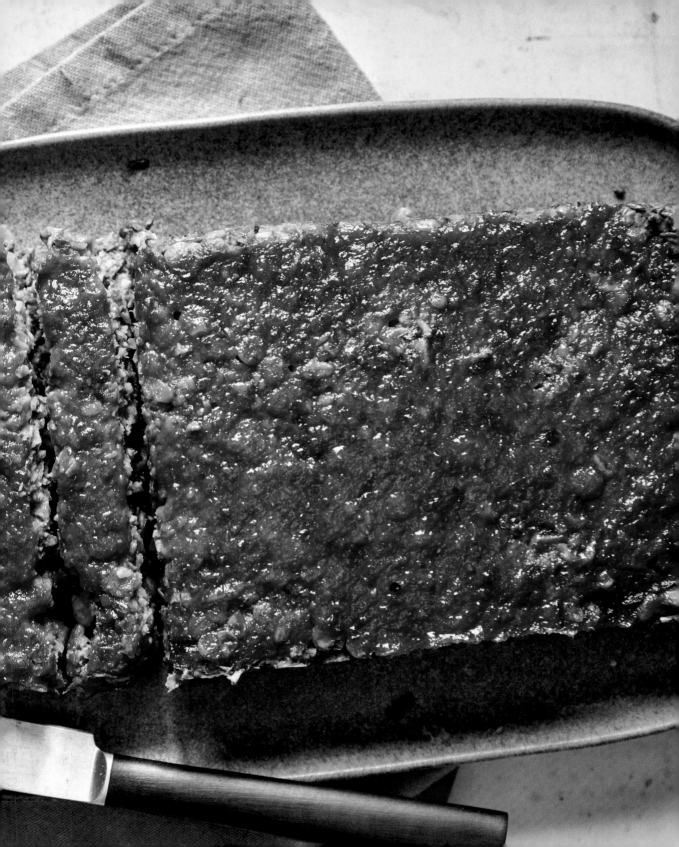

Pesto Farro Risotto

with Snap Peas and Asparagus

PREP TIME// 15 minutes

COOK TIME// 1 hour

SERVES// 4

3 tablespoons avocado oil

1 medium leek, cleaned and
thinly sliced

3 garlic cloves, minced

1 tablespoon fresh thyme

1½ cups farro, rinsed

Sea salt and freshly ground black
pepper to taste

½ cup dry white wine

4 cups low-sodium vegetable stock

1 pound asparagus, trimmed and cut
into 1-inch pieces

6 ounces sugar snap peas, cut in half
(about 2 cups)

½ cup Almond Parmesan, plus
additional to garnish (page 241)

1 recipe Pea and Pumpkin Seed Pesto
(page 245)

2 tablespoons chopped fresh basil,
to garnish

2 tablespoons chopped fresh flat-leaf
parsley, to garnish

Risotto is often intimidating because it takes a lot of time as well as skill to cook the rice perfectly by adding small amounts of stock at a time. This farro risotto is my foolproof and whole grain take on a traditional risotto. The stock is added all at one time and the farro simmered until it becomes the creamy consistency of risotto. Of course, I wanted to keep the traditional flavors of wine and cheese (thanks, nutritional yeast!) plus add a twist of pesto to make for an elegant crowd-pleasing recipe.

1 In a large Dutch oven or heavy-bottomed pot, heat the avocado oil over medium-high heat. Add the leek and garlic and allow to cook for about 4 minutes, or until softened. Add the thyme and farro and allow to toast for another minute. Season with salt and pepper.

2 Deglaze the pan with white wine (see Tip) and simmer for about 5 minutes, or until reduced by half. Add the stock, season again with salt and pepper, and simmer partially covered for 40 to 45 minutes, stirring occasionally, until the farro is cooked and the risotto has thickened. If the stock reduces but the farro is not fully cooked, add up to 1 cup of water and continue simmering. During the last 5 to 10 minutes of cooking, add the asparagus and the sugar snap peas. Add additional stock or water if the risotto is too thick.

3 Stir in the parm. Divide among four bowls and swirl a spoonful of the pesto through the risotto. Garnish with more parm, basil, and parsley and serve.

TIP: When you deglaze a pan, you add a small amount of wine (or stock) after browning veggies, spices, or protein. Be sure to scrape up any of the browned bits off the bottom of the pot. This is where all the flavor is! By reducing the wine by half before adding additional cooking liquid, you are concentrating that delicious flavor, which will really highlight the spring veggies in this recipe.

Gwen Jorgenson's Tortilla de Patatas (Spanish Potato Omelet)

ATHLETE RECIPE: Gwen Jorgenson is an American distance runner and former professional triathlete. She is the 2016 Rio Olympic Champion in the triathlon. She is also the 2014 and 2015 ITU World Triathlon Series Champion. Gwen's husband, Patrick Lemieux, is a chef (and former pro cyclist) and helps Gwen fuel for her training. His cooking was especially helpful during the nine months she spent breastfeeding and working herself back into shape postpartum.

"Tortilla de Patatas is served at every café in Vitoria-Gasteiz in the Basque region of Spain, where I lived and trained for four years leading up to my Olympic Gold in Rio. On my way home from swim practice, I loved stopping at a café for a slice of this potato omelet. I enjoyed it so much that my husband, Patrick, and I asked our favorite Basque chef to teach us how to make it. This potato omelet is a super easy recipe and perfect for breakfast, lunch, or dinner or as a snack."

PREP TIME// 10 minutes
COOK TIME// 20 minutes
SERVES// 2

3 large russet potatoes, peeled and chopped into ½-inch pieces (about 3 cups)

5 tablespoons extra-virgin olive oil, plus additional as needed

Sea salt and freshly ground black pepper to taste

6 large eggs

1 In a large bowl, toss the potatoes with 3 tablespoons of the olive oil. Transfer the potatoes to a 10-inch nonstick sauté pan over medium heat. Allow to cook slowly, 8 to 10 minutes, shaking the pan every few minutes, until almost tender (the potatoes shouldn't brown until they are almost finished). Season with salt and pepper.

2 In a large bowl, whisk the eggs one at a time, then season with salt and pepper. When the potatoes are finished, add them to the bowl with the eggs and quickly stir to combine. Return the sauté pan to medium heat and add the remaining 2 tablespoons oil. Pour the egg-and-potato mixture back into the sauté pan and cook slowly, occasionally scraping toward the center to create a wall around the edge. Cover and cook for 6 to 7 minutes, until the middle is just set. Remove from the heat. Place a plate on top of the pan and quickly flip the pan upside down to transfer the omelet to the plate. Serve.

Kara Goucher's Chili-Spiced Salmon

with Mango Salsa

ATHLETE RECIPE: Kara Goucher is a two-time Olympian and Track and Field World Championship silver medalist. She loves to cook and fuel her and her family's bodies with real whole foods. She worked closely with Lottie in 2015, leading up to the Olympic marathon trials. During this time, Lottie lived with the Gouchers to focus on Kara's nutrition and optimize her performance. Lottie continues to collaborate with Kara and speaks at her annual retreat training camp.

"I love to eat this salmon for dinner the night before a hard workout session. It fuels my body with good protein and lots of healthy fats. As an endurance athlete, I serve it with coconut rice to make a complete meal. Plus, it's a real winner with my husband and son and has become a favorite recipe in our home."

1 **For the Mango Salsa:** In a medium bowl, combine the mango, onion, bell pepper, jalapeño, cilantro, and lime juice. Season with salt and set aside to marinate while you prepare the fish.

2 **For the Chili-Spiced Salmon:** Preheat the oven to 400°F. Line a baking sheet with parchment paper.

3 In a small bowl, mix together the garlic powder, onion powder, paprika, chili powder, cumin, and salt.

4 Place the fish fillets on the prepared baking sheet and sprinkle each one with the spice rub. Bake for 15 to 20 minutes on the middle rack, until the fish is opaque, cooked through, and flakes easily with a fork.

5 Place the fillets on a serving plate and top with the mango salsa. Serve with coconut rice, if desired.

TIP: I like to double this spice rub to have on hand for other proteins and vegetables as an easy weeknight meal.

PREP TIME// 15 minutes
COOK TIME// 20 minutes
SERVES// 4

Mango Salsa

1 mango, pit removed, peeled, and diced

½ medium red onion, finely diced

½ red bell pepper, cored, seeded, and diced small

1 jalapeño, seeded and finely diced

½ cup chopped fresh cilantro

2 tablespoons fresh lime juice

Sea salt to taste

Chili-Spiced Salmon

1 teaspoon garlic powder

1 teaspoon onion powder

1 teaspoon sweet paprika

1 teaspoon chili powder

½ teaspoon ground cumin

½ teaspoon sea salt

4 (4- to 6-ounce) skin-on salmon fillets

Coconut rice, to serve (optional)

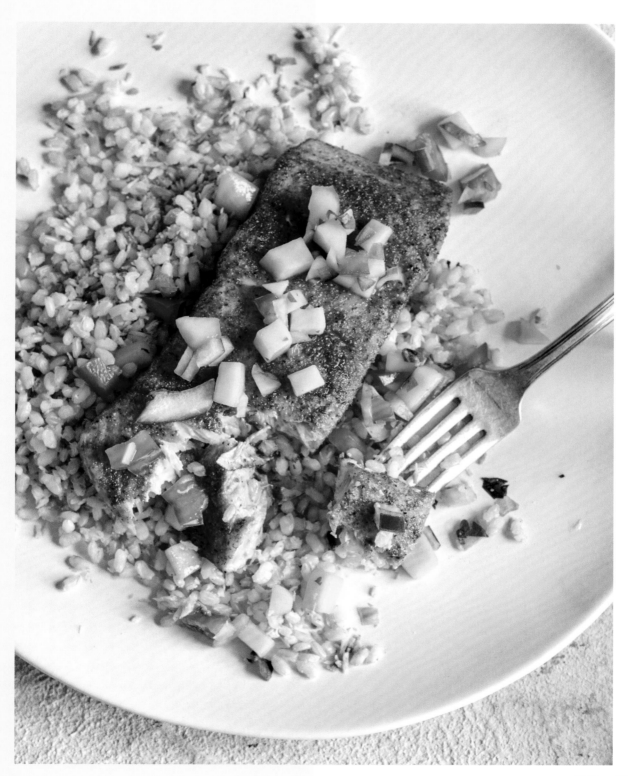

Linsey Corbin's Beet Burger

ATHLETE RECIPE: Linsey Corbin is a professional triathlete who lives and trains in her hometown of Bend, Oregon. She is an eight-time Ironman champion and has received top American honors at both the Ironman and 70.3 World Championship events. In the summer of 2014, Linsey set a new Ironman American record with the fifth-fastest time in the history of the sport. Linsey studied exercise physiology at the University of Montana and has always had a passion for sports nutrition and learning how fueling the body well leads to great performances. When she's not racing and training, Linsey enjoys spending time with her husband, Chris, and their golden retriever, Chimmy.

"These beet burgers are inspired by a meal made at a training camp in Tucson a couple of years ago. My friend Heather Jackson made her recipe for a beet-quinoa burger, and I liked them so much I had to make my own. Even if you're not a fan of beets, give these a try. My husband, Chris, is not a beet lover, but now this is one of his favorite veg-friendly dinners. These burgers are hearty and nutrient dense, perfect for after a big training day. I like to eat mine either on a bun or over a salad with hummus and veggies."

1 In a large sauté pan, heat 2 tablespoons of the olive oil over medium heat. Add the onion and cook for 5 minutes, or until softened. Add the mushrooms, season with salt and pepper, and cook for another 5 minutes, or until the mushrooms soften. Remove from the heat and allow to cool slightly.

2 In a large bowl, mash the black beans with a fork or potato masher. Add the cooled onion and mushrooms, the quinoa, beets, cumin, chili powder, and paprika and stir to combine. Season with salt and pepper.

3 Add the oats and fold until just incorporated. Form the mixture into six to eight 1-inch-thick patties. If the mixture seems too wet, add a few more oats. Place the patties on a plate, cover with plastic wrap, and refrigerate for 2 hours or up to overnight to set.

4 When ready to cook, preheat the oven to 375°F.

5 Take the patties out of the refrigerator and allow them to sit at room temperature for 20 minutes. Grease a large baking sheet with the remaining 1 tablespoon oil. Arrange the patties on the prepared baking sheet and bake on the middle rack for 30 to 40 minutes, flipping halfway through, until golden brown and cooked through.

6 Serve on buns and garnish with any or all of the suggested toppings.

TIP: Feel free to freeze these patties after cooking and cooling to save for another busy weeknight meal. Just thaw the burgers and reheat in the oven or in a sauté pan on the stove.

PREP TIME// 25 minutes + 2 hours refrigeration or up to overnight
COOK TIME// 50 minutes
SERVES// 6 to 8

3 tablespoons extra-virgin olive oil

½ yellow onion, diced small

4 or 5 button mushrooms, chopped

Sea salt and freshly ground black pepper to taste

1 (15-ounce) can black beans, drained and rinsed

½ cup cooked quinoa

2 to 3 small beets, peeled and grated (about 1 cup)

1 teaspoon ground cumin

½ teaspoon chili powder or red chili flakes

½ teaspoon smoked paprika (optional)

½ cup old-fashioned rolled oats or almond meal

6 to 8 whole wheat hamburger buns

Optional Toppings

Small handful of greens like lettuce, spinach, or arugula

1 to 2 large tomatoes, sliced

1 to 2 avocados, pitted, peeled, and thinly sliced

Mustard, to serve

Hummus, to serve

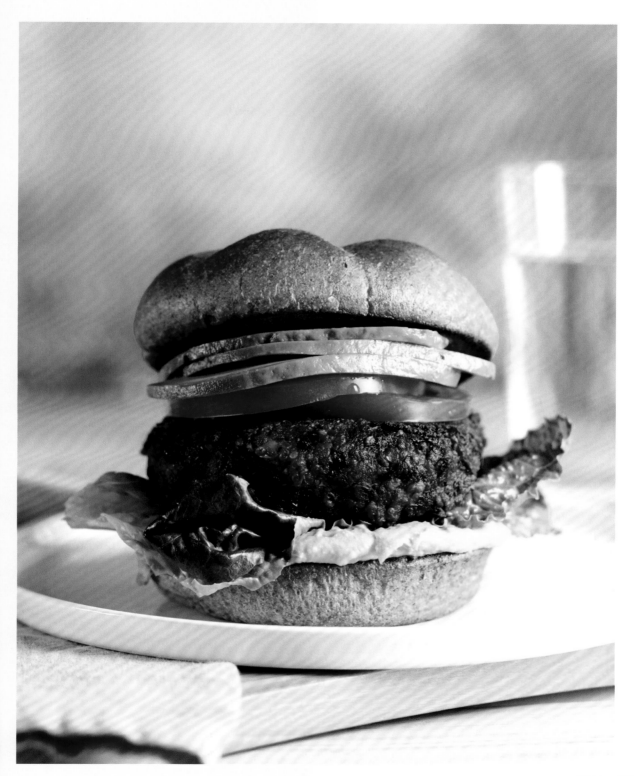

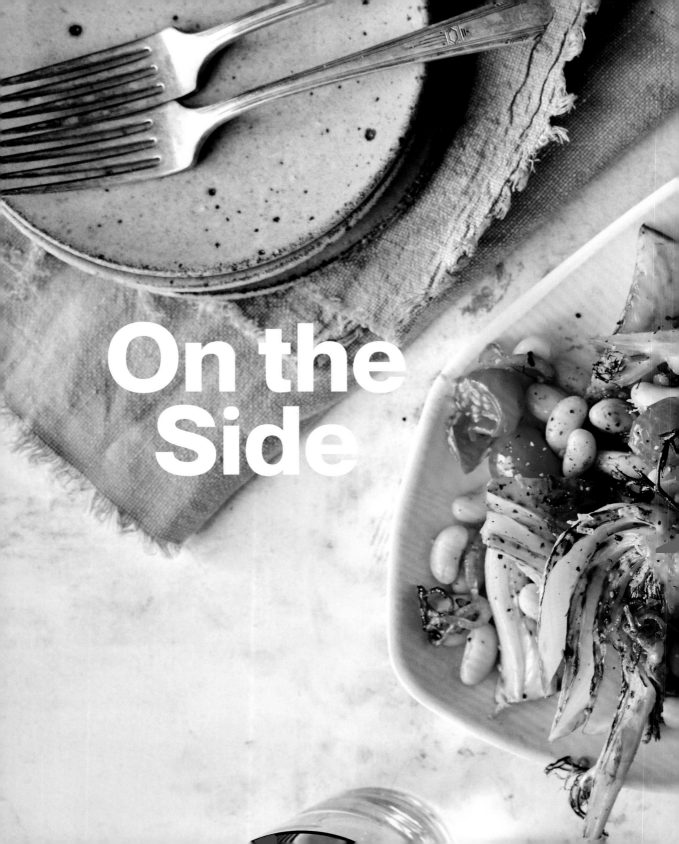

On the
Side

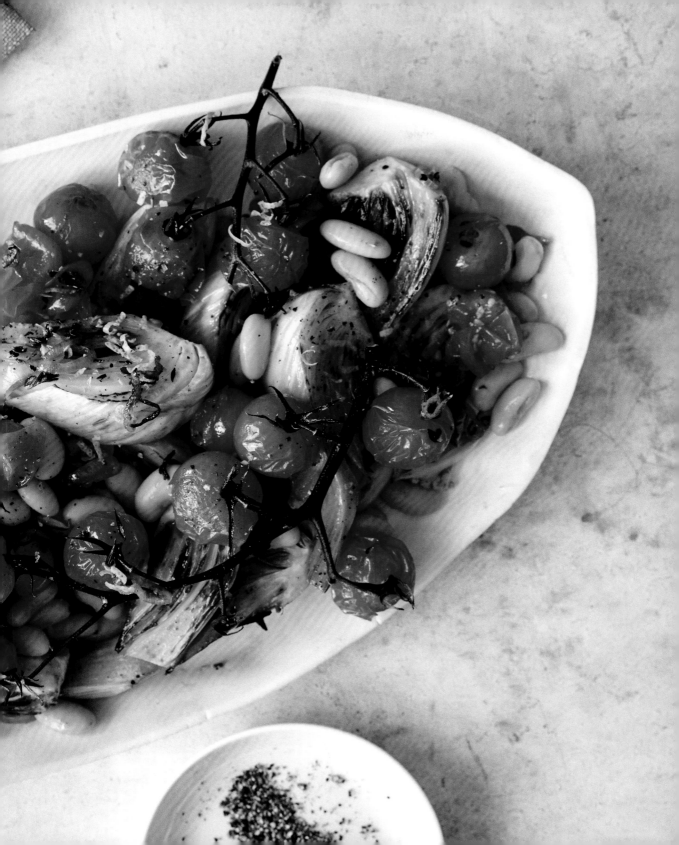

Side dishes are always a highlight for me—there are so many times at home or when eating at a restaurant that I'll just make or order a couple of sides as my main course. Sides let you have variety and add something to any menu to make the whole meal complete. The side recipes in this chapter pair well with other dishes in the book but can also stand alone as a main course or be combined with other sides for a tapas-style dinner.

One unique side that I had to include was my Braised Apple Dijon Cabbage (page 159). Cabbage isn't everyone's favorite veggie, but try this recipe and you will never look at humble cabbage the same! My Farro Corn Bread (page 154) is a recipe based off a favorite former restaurant of mine—I've been wanting to create my own version for years, and I must say I love it both as a side and a snack. Lastly, the Vegan Mexican Street Corn (page 150) is a recipe that keeps me smiling every time I make it. It's something I always order alongside a taco when I get the chance, so I knew I had to come up with a plant-based version.

Vegan Mexican Street Corn

PREP TIME// 10 minutes
COOK TIME// 20 minutes
SERVES// 6

Avocado Sauce

1 avocado, pitted and peeled

2 tablespoons fresh lime juice

½ cup hot water (115°F to 120°F)

Sea salt to taste

Grilled Corn

¼ cup avocado oil

1 teaspoon chili powder

1 teaspoon smoked paprika

Sea salt to taste

6 ears corn, shucked

¼ cup Almond Parmesan (page 241)

½ cup chopped fresh cilantro, to garnish

Lime wedges, to serve

Although I live in New York City, I travel frequently to Los Angeles for work, which gives me the opportunity to explore tacos in different places. This street corn is always the side dish I order because of its smoky, charred, and cheesy flavors. Here, I transform this flavorful corn into a vegan, dairy-free version that is still full of these vibrant flavors.

1 **For the Avocado Sauce:** Place the avocado into a high-speed blender or mini food processor. Add the lime juice and hot water and blend until smooth. Season with salt and set aside.

2 **For the Grilled Corn:** Preheat a grill or grill pan to medium-high heat.

3 In a small bowl, whisk together the avocado oil, chili powder, and paprika and season with salt.

4 Place the corn on the grill and cook for 5 to 6 minutes per side, until charred. Remove to a platter. Brush the hot corn with the avocado oil mixture. Sprinkle the corn on all sides with the "parm." Drizzle with the avocado sauce and garnish with cilantro. Serve with lime wedges.

TIP: The same oil and spice mixture that's used on the grilled corn can also be used to sear other vegetables and your favorite protein for a smoky, spicy flavor.

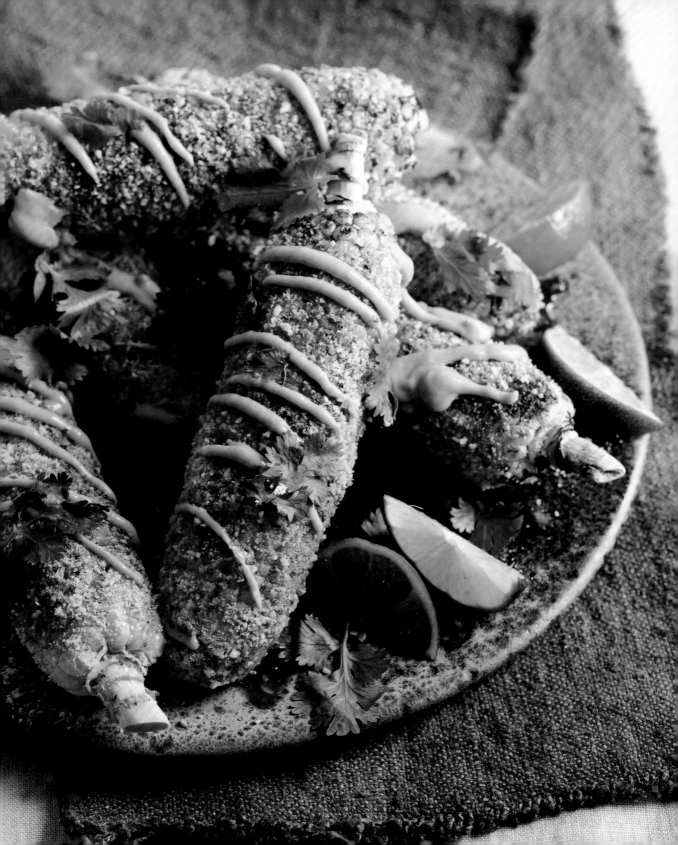

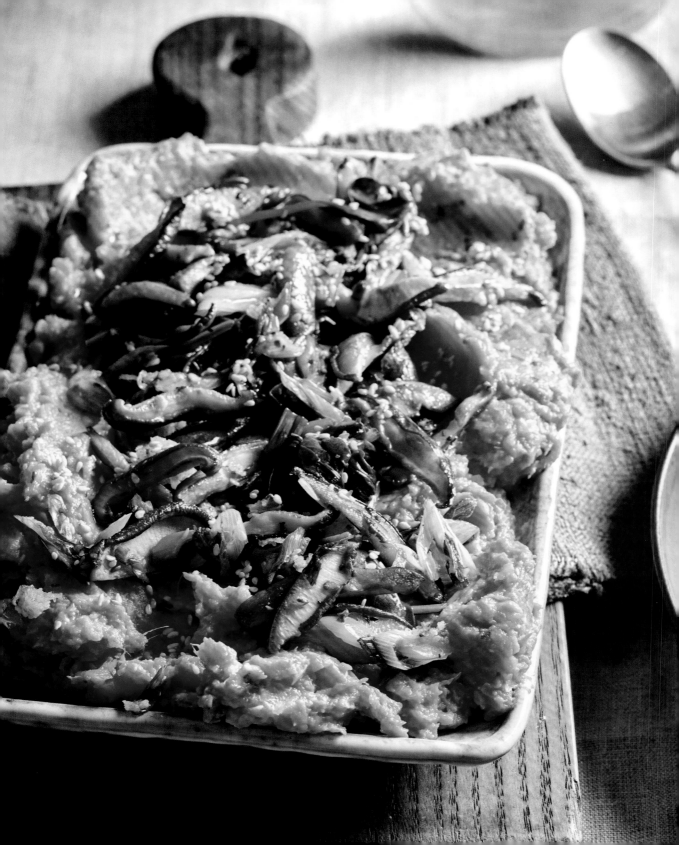

Miso-Mashed Sweet Potatoes

with Ginger Shiitakes

PREP TIME// 15 minutes

COOK TIME// 25 minutes

SERVES// 4

Optional Mushroom Topping

2 tablespoons avocado oil

2 scallions (white and light green parts), thinly sliced, plus additional to garnish

2 garlic cloves, minced

1 (1-inch) piece of ginger, peeled and grated

1 (5-ounce) container sliced shiitake mushrooms

2 cups packed baby spinach

Sea salt to taste

Sweet Potatoes

2 pounds sweet potatoes, peeled and cut into 1-inch cubes

2 tablespoons white or yellow miso paste

2 scallions (white and light green parts), minced, plus additional sliced to garnish

¼ cup unsweetened nut milk

Sea salt to taste

1 tablespoon toasted sesame seeds

Miso, what is it? You've probably seen this ingredient on a restaurant menu or in a food magazine and wondered what it was and how to use it. Miso is fermented soybean paste. It's great for the digestive system and provides healthy gut bacteria. Additionally, the fermentation of miso helps you absorb the nutrients from the soybeans better. This is important because soybeans are a good source of protein and contain all the amino acids needed for your health. When cooking with miso, keep in mind a little goes a long way! The flavor adds a boost of umami and salt to any dish. It's the perfect complement to the natural sweetness of sweet potatoes in this recipe.

1 **For the Optional Mushroom Topping:** In a large sauté pan, heat the avocado oil over medium-high heat. Add the scallions, garlic, and ginger and cook for a minute, until fragrant. Add the mushrooms and cook for about 6 minutes, or until lightly golden and tender. Season with salt to taste. Add the baby spinach and allow to just wilt, then remove from the heat. Cover to keep warm.

2 **For the Sweet Potatoes:** Place the sweet potatoes in a large pot and cover with salted water. Bring to a boil, then reduce the heat and allow to simmer for 15 to 18 minutes, until very tender.

3 Drain the potatoes and mash using a potato masher. Stir in the miso paste, scallions, and nut milk, and season with salt to taste.

4 Transfer the mashed sweet potato to a serving bowl and garnish with sesame seeds and scallions. Top with the mushrooms, if desired, and serve.

Farro Corn Bread

PREP TIME// 5 minutes

COOK TIME// 42 minutes

SERVES// 9

¼ cup coconut oil, melted, plus additional for greasing the pan

½ cup old-fashioned rolled oats

1 cup yellow cornmeal

½ cup oat flour

1 tablespoon ground flaxseed

½ teaspoon baking soda

½ teaspoon baking powder

½ teaspoon sea salt

1 cup unsweetened apple juice

½ cup unsweetened applesauce

½ cup cooked and cooled farro or other whole grain

¼ cup frozen corn kernels, thawed

1 tablespoon raw sesame seeds

Optional Tahini Miso Butter

¼ cup tahini, well stirred

1 tablespoon plus 1 teaspoon white or yellow miso paste

Fruit-sweetened jam, to serve (optional)

Inspired by the corn bread recipe from Angelica's Kitchen, an iconic vegan restaurant formerly in NYC, this corn bread is a simple and delicious side to add to any meal. Angelica's Kitchen uses brown rice in their corn bread, but I chose farro for its extra nutty flavor. I also stir in corn kernels for some fresh texture. Try serving with the tahini miso "butter" and jam. This corn bread is the perfect accompaniment for my Southwestern Vegetable Slow Cooker Chili (page 94).

1 Preheat the oven to 350°F. Grease an 8 × 8-inch baking dish with coconut oil and line with parchment paper, allowing the sides to overhang as handles.

2 In a large bowl, stir together the oats, cornmeal, flour, flaxseed, baking soda, baking powder, and salt. In a medium bowl, whisk together the apple juice, applesauce, and coconut oil. Make a well in the dry ingredients and add the apple juice mixture to the center of the well. Stir gently to combine. Add the farro and corn kernels and fold until just incorporated.

3 Scrape the batter into the prepared baking dish and sprinkle with sesame seeds. Bake for 38 to 42 minutes, until an inserted toothpick comes out clean. If the corn bread is getting too brown, lightly place a piece of foil over the top. Allow to cool for 30 minutes in the pan before slicing and serving.

4 **For the Optional Tahini Miso Butter:** In a small bowl, stir together the tahini and miso paste until smooth and combined. Serve with jam, if desired, alongside the corn bread.

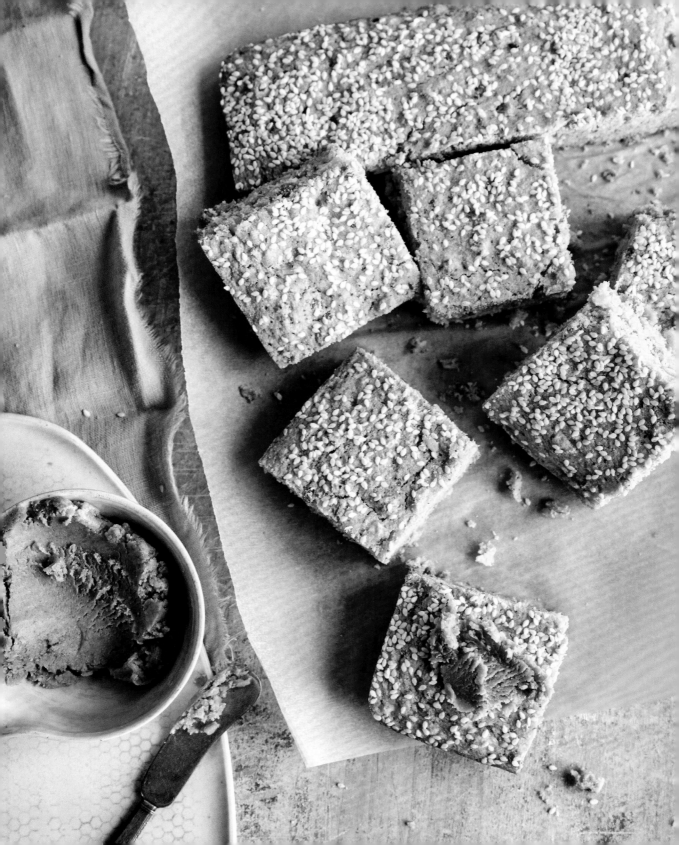

Lemon Anchovy Broccolini

PREP TIME// 10 minutes

COOK TIME// 15 minutes

SERVES// 4

2 tablespoons avocado oil

1 medium red onion, thinly sliced

1 pound broccolini, cut into
2-inch pieces

Sea salt and freshly ground black
pepper to taste

2 garlic cloves, thinly sliced

2 to 3 anchovies, or 1 to 2 teaspoons
anchovy paste

Pinch of red chili flakes (optional)

¼ cup water

1 tablespoon capers, drained

1 lemon, zested and juiced

2 tablespoons roasted and salted
sunflower seeds

As one of my favorite side dishes to add to any protein or meal, this broccolini has a nice tang with a hint of spice and garlic. It also has a natural saltiness from the anchovies, which also boast so many healthy qualities. Anchovies are rich in iron, which is a mineral important for athletes since it helps produce hemoglobin and myoglobin, which transport oxygen through the body and to the muscles.

1 In a large cast-iron skillet or heavy-bottomed sauté pan, heat the avocado oil over medium-high heat. Add the onion and allow to cook for 3 to 4 minutes, until softened. Add the broccolini and cook for 5 minutes, or until just wilted. Season with salt and pepper.

2 Add the garlic, anchovies, and chili flakes (if using) and cook for another minute, or until the anchovies dissolve. Deglaze the pan with the water and simmer for 4 to 5 minutes, until the broccolini is tender.

3 During the last minute of cooking, sprinkle in the capers, add the lemon zest and lemon juice, and top with sunflower seeds. Season with additional salt and pepper, if necessary.

Chili-Spiced Crispy Brussels Sprouts

PREP TIME// 10 minutes

COOK TIME// 30 minutes

SERVES// 4

1 pound Brussels sprouts, trimmed and cut in half or quartered if large

½ bunch scallions (white and light green parts), thinly sliced

3 garlic cloves, minced

2 pitted Medjool dates, chopped

2 tablespoons avocado oil

Sea salt to taste and freshly ground black pepper

¼ cup rice wine vinegar

1 tablespoon liquid aminos (I like Bragg)

1 tablespoon sriracha

2 tablespoons toasted sesame seeds

Lime wedges, to serve

Crispy, spicy Brussels sprouts have become a restaurant trend over the past few years, so I was inspired to make my own. I like to oven-roast my Brussels sprouts until golden brown and then toss them in a tangy and spicy sauce. The chopped dates add for a fun, sweet surprise that complements the vibrant sauce nicely.

1 Preheat the oven to 425°F. Line a baking sheet with parchment paper.

2 On the prepared baking sheet, toss together the Brussels sprouts, scallions, garlic, dates, and avocado oil. Season with salt and pepper. Roast for 25 to 30 minutes, tossing halfway through, until golden brown and crispy.

3 Meanwhile, in a small bowl, whisk together the vinegar, liquid aminos, sriracha, and sesame seeds. During the last 5 minutes of cooking, pour the sauce over the Brussels sprouts and toss to evenly coat. Return the Brussels sprouts to the oven to heat the sauce through.

4 Season with salt again, if necessary, and serve with lime wedges.

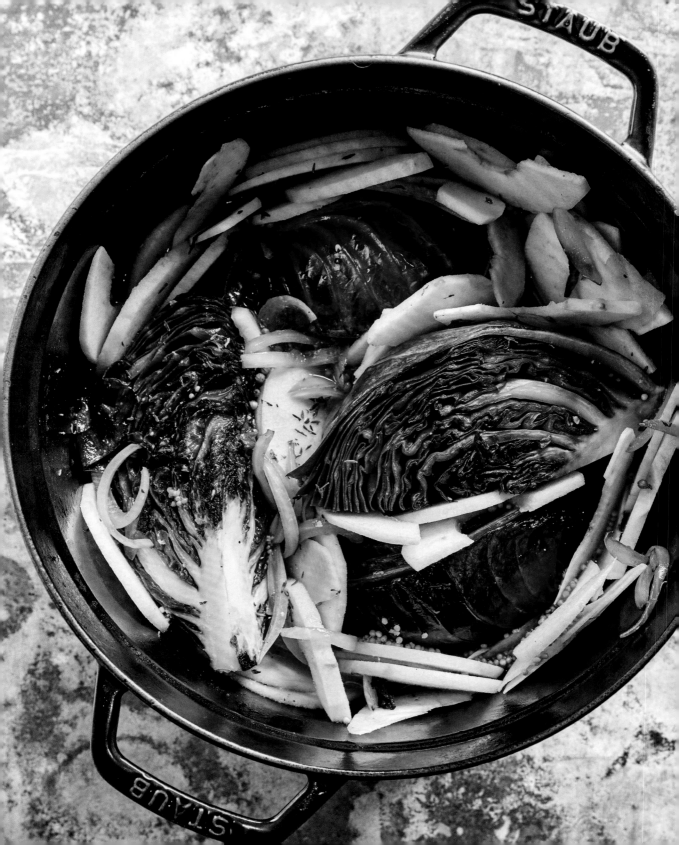

Braised Apple Dijon Cabbage

PREP TIME// 10 minutes

COOK TIME// 50 minutes

SERVES// 4

2 tablespoons avocado oil

Small head of red cabbage,
cut into 4 wedges

1 small yellow onion, thinly sliced

1 teaspoon dried thyme

½ teaspoon coriander seed

½ teaspoon mustard seed

2 medium Granny Smith apples,
peeled and sliced

Sea salt and freshly ground black
pepper, to serve

2 cups low-sodium vegetable stock,
plus additional as needed

3 tablespoons apple cider vinegar

2 tablespoons Dijon mustard

¼ cup chopped fresh flat-leaf parsley,
to garnish

Braised cabbage has always been on my recipe inspiration to-do list. It's a gourmet recipe using minimal, inexpensive ingredients. I like to add it to a holiday menu because it pairs so nicely with all the other mains and side dishes on the table and is also easy to make. I add apples to my version as a natural sweetness that works nicely with the hearty cabbage, tangy vinegar, and spicy Dijon.

1 In a large Dutch oven or heavy-bottomed pot, heat the avocado oil over medium-high heat. Add the cabbage and cook for 7 to 10 minutes, until the cabbage is lightly browned on both sides. Add the onion halfway through the cooking of the cabbage and cook until softened. Add the thyme, coriander seed, mustard seed, and apples and cook another minute. (Depending on how large your Dutch oven is, you may need to remove one-quarter of the cabbage to a plate to evenly distribute the spices and apples. Return the cabbage to the pot once distributed.) Season with salt and pepper.

2 Deglaze the pot with the stock, scraping any browned bits up from the bottom of the pan (the stock should come about halfway up the cabbage). Bring to a boil, then reduce to a simmer and partially cover the pot. Simmer for 30 to 35 minutes, until the cabbage is very tender. Add more stock if the pot becomes dry.

3 Once tender, shut off the heat and remove one-quarter of the cabbage to a plate. Whisk the vinegar and mustard into the cooking liquid. Return the cabbage to the pot and season again with salt and pepper if necessary. Garnish with parsley and serve.

Cauliflower Mujadara

PREP TIME// 5 minutes

COOK TIME// 15 minutes

SERVES// 4

2 tablespoons avocado oil

1 large white onion, diced

3 garlic cloves, minced

1 teaspoon cumin seed

½ teaspoon dried oregano

Pinch of red chili flakes (optional)

Sea salt and freshly ground black pepper to taste

2 cups cooked brown lentils, cooled

6 cups cauliflower rice

Mujadara is a classic Middle Eastern dish using rice, lentils, and caramelized onions. Inspired by my family's Middle Eastern roots, my mom often made this for dinner when I was growing up. In my version, I decided to use cauliflower rice to make the recipe plant forward. The caramelized onions are key to adding a rich, slightly sweet flavor. It's the perfect weeknight side dish or base to a rice, protein, and veggie bowl.

In a large heavy-bottomed pot or Dutch oven, heat the avocado oil over medium-high heat. Add the onion and cook for 6 to 7 minutes, stirring occasionally, until golden. Add the garlic, cumin seed, oregano, and chili flakes (if using), and toast for another minute. Season with salt and pepper. Add the lentils and cauliflower rice and cook for 5 to 6 minutes, stirring frequently, until tender and combined. Season again with salt and pepper and serve.

Roasted Garlic
Green Hummus

PREP TIME // 15 minutes

COOK TIME // 45 minutes

SERVES // 4 to 6

Roasted Garlic

Head of garlic, top cut off

1 tablespoon avocado oil

Hummus

2 (15-ounce) can chickpeas, drained and rinsed

½ cup roughly chopped fresh flat-leaf parsley, plus additional to garnish

½ cup roughly chopped fresh chives, plus additional to garnish

6 tablespoons fresh lemon juice

½ cup tahini, well stirred

⅓ cup extra-virgin olive oil, plus 1 tablespoon additional to serve

Sea salt to taste

½ cup hot water (115°F to 120°F), as needed

4 whole wheat pita, warmed, to serve

Carrot sticks, bell pepper, and cucumber slices, to serve

Who doesn't love a good hummus? It's great as the bottom of a grain bowl, on a sandwich or salad, or even just by itself with whole wheat pita or veggies as a snack. What I love about this hummus is the addition of roasted garlic. Roasting the garlic brings out a sweet and more subtle flavor that makes the hummus so flavorful and creamy. And garlic has many health benefits, like boosting the immune system with vitamin C and reducing cholesterol and blood pressure.

1 **For the Roasted Garlic:** Preheat the oven to 400°F.

2 Place the head of garlic on a piece of foil, drizzle with the avocado oil, and wrap tightly. Place on a baking sheet and roast for 35 to 45 minutes, until fragrant and caramelized. Allow to cool completely. Once cooled, squeeze the cloves out into a bowl and set aside.

3 **For the Hummus:** Place ¼ cup of the chickpeas in a small bowl and set aside. In the bowl of a food processor fitted with the blade attachment, blend the remaining chickpeas, parsley, chives, lemon juice, tahini, and the roasted garlic cloves until smooth. While the machine is running, slowly stream in the olive oil until combined. Season with salt. Add some hot water to adjust the consistency, if necessary. The hummus should be super smooth but not too thick.

4 Transfer the hummus to a serving bowl and drizzle with 1 tablespoon olive oil. Garnish with parsley, chives, and the reserved whole chickpeas. Serve with pita and veggies. Store in an airtight container in the refrigerator for up to 4 days.

Hasselback Sweet Potatoes

with Mustard Seed and Yogurt

PREP TIME// 15 minutes

COOK TIME// 50 minutes

SERVES// 4

4 medium sweet potatoes, scrubbed

¼ cup avocado oil

2 teaspoons chopped fresh thyme

2 teaspoons chopped fresh rosemary

½ teaspoon ground cinnamon

Pinch of cayenne pepper (optional)

Sea salt and freshly ground black pepper to taste

1 tablespoon mustard seeds

½ cup plain coconut yogurt, to garnish (optional)

2 teaspoons thinly sliced fresh chives, to garnish

2 teaspoons chopped fresh flat-leaf parsley, to garnish

These potatoes are so simple but look so much more complicated. The hasselback technique allows for the base of the potato to cook until tender, while the individual potato slices form crispy tops, making for a soft but crunchy texture all in the same bite. I first tried these potatoes several years ago when visiting a family friend in London, and while that recipe used russet potatoes, I wanted to put my spin on it, by using sweet potatoes here.

1 Preheat the oven to 400°F. Line a prepared baking sheet with parchment paper.

2 Slice each sweet potato crosswise into ¼-inch-thick slices, being careful not to cut through the potato completely—there needs to be a base so the sweet potato can stand.

3 In a small bowl, combine the avocado oil, thyme, rosemary, cinnamon, cayenne (if using), and salt and pepper to taste. Rub all over the outside of the potatoes and in between the slices. Sprinkle the potatoes with the mustard seeds. Bake for 45 to 50 minutes, fanning out the sweet potato slices with a fork halfway through baking. The sweet potatoes should be tender when finished baking with crispy tops on the hasselback slices.

4 Garnish with yogurt (if using), chives, and parsley.

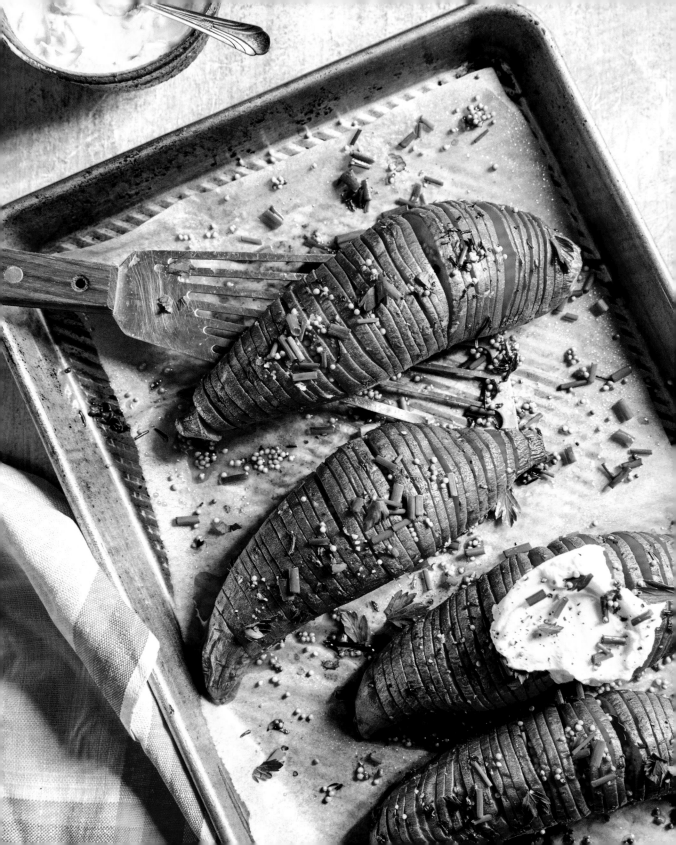

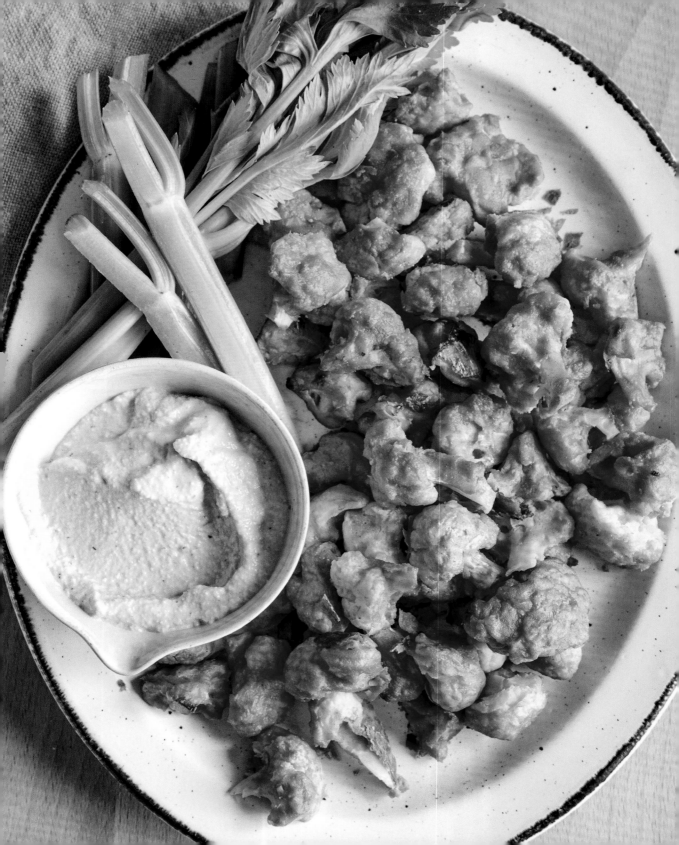

Buffalo
Cauliflower Wings

PREP TIME// 10 minutes

COOK TIME// 50 minutes

SERVES// 4 to 6

Avocado oil cooking spray, for greasing (I use a Misto)

1 cup chickpea flour

¾ cup water

2 teaspoons garlic powder

1½ teaspoons sweet paprika

Sea salt to taste

Large head cauliflower (3½ to 4 pounds), cut into small florets (about 10 cups florets)

⅓ cup favorite hot sauce (I like Frank's RedHot)

1 tablespoon avocado oil

2 tablespoons chopped fresh flat-leaf parsley, to garnish

1 recipe Vegan Ranch Dressing (page 237), to serve

This is a great appetizer for any party, as it's always a crowd-pleaser. Here, I use chickpea flour as the gluten-free breading substitute since it's high in antioxidants as well as vitamins and minerals like folate. Chickpea flour is also quite filling and has fewer carbs than white flour, so it keeps your blood sugar at a lower level.

1   Preheat the oven to 425°F. Line two baking sheets with parchment paper and grease with the avocado oil spray.

2   In a large bowl, whisk together the flour, water, garlic powder, and paprika and season with salt. Be sure the mixture can nicely coat the cauliflower but isn't too thick.

3   Toss the cauliflower florets in the batter to coat evenly and divide between the two prepared baking sheets. (Be sure not to overcrowd the baking sheets so the cauliflower browns and doesn't steam!) Place in the oven to roast for 20 minutes.

4   Meanwhile, in a small bowl, whisk together the hot sauce and avocado oil. Remove the cauliflower from the oven and drizzle the hot sauce over it. Toss to lightly coat the cauliflower. Return the baking sheets to the oven and bake another 25 to 30 minutes, until lightly golden and crunchy.

5   Garnish the cauliflower with parsley and serve with the dressing on the side.

TIP: Roasting 101. Never crowd your baking sheet! The vegetables must have space in between to allow for even browning rather than steaming.

Balsamic and Thyme Roasted Mushrooms

PREP TIME// 15 minutes

COOK TIME// 25 minutes

SERVES// 4

¼ cup balsamic vinegar

2 tablespoons avocado oil

1 teaspoon dried thyme

1 pound cremini mushrooms, halved or quartered if large

¾ pound shiitake mushrooms, stems removed

Sea salt and freshly ground black pepper to taste

2 cups cooked brown rice, to serve (optional)

When I'm planning dinner, I like to have some easy side dishes that complete a meal but aren't too complicated or time consuming. Roasted mushrooms with a simple balsamic and thyme marinade is often my solution. They are full of flavor but still let me focus on preparing the main course. With the leftovers, I often reheat, place over brown rice and greens, and make a fried egg to go on top for another complete meal.

1 Preheat the oven to 425°F. Line a rimmed baking sheet with parchment paper.

2 In a small bowl, whisk together the vinegar, avocado oil, and thyme. Place the mushrooms in a large bowl and pour the vinaigrette over them. Season with salt and pepper and toss to evenly coat.

3 Spread evenly onto the prepared baking sheet. Roast for 20 to 25 minutes, until golden brown and tender. Serve over brown rice, if desired. Mushrooms can be kept in an airtight container in the refrigerator for up to 3 days.

TIP: The best way to clean your mushrooms is by brushing off the dirt with a dry paper towel or pastry brush.

Braised Swiss Chard and Kabocha Squash

PREP TIME// 15 minutes

COOK TIME// 40 minutes

SERVES// 4

2 tablespoons avocado oil

1 shallot, diced

3 garlic cloves, minced

2 teaspoons ground mustard

1 teaspoon ground coriander

1 kabocha squash (about 2½ pounds), seeded, and cut into 1-inch-thick wedges

3 pitted Medjool dates, chopped

Sea salt and freshly ground black pepper to taste

3 cups low-sodium vegetable stock

8 ounces Swiss chard, chopped (about 6 cups)

1 navel orange, zested and juiced

1 tablespoon apple cider vinegar

This dish always "wows" family and friends; the great news is, it's just a couple of steps that all come together in under an hour. The flavors blend together well with the richness of the squash and Swiss chard, the sweetness from the dates, and the hint of acid from the orange and vinegar as the finishing touch. It's one of my signature winter recipes to make as a side dish or a main course.

1   In a large Dutch oven or heavy-bottomed pot, heat the avocado oil over medium-high heat. Add the shallot and garlic and cook about 4 minutes, or until softened. Add the mustard and coriander and toast for another minute. Add the squash and dates and season with salt and pepper.

2   Deglaze the pan with the stock and bring to a simmer. Allow to simmer for 15 to 20 minutes, partially covered, adding the Swiss chard during the last 10 minutes of cooking. The squash should be tender and the liquid stewed and reduced by half.

3   Stir in the orange zest, orange juice, and vinegar and serve.

TIP: Adding a touch of vinegar or citrus at the end of a rich vegetable or protein stew dish helps highlight the natural flavors and sweetness of each individual ingredient in a recipe.

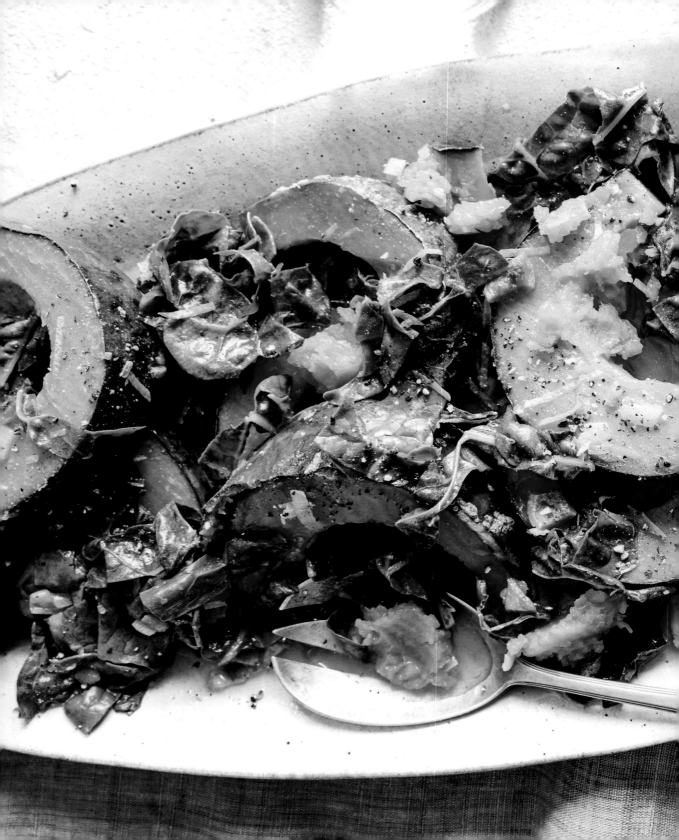

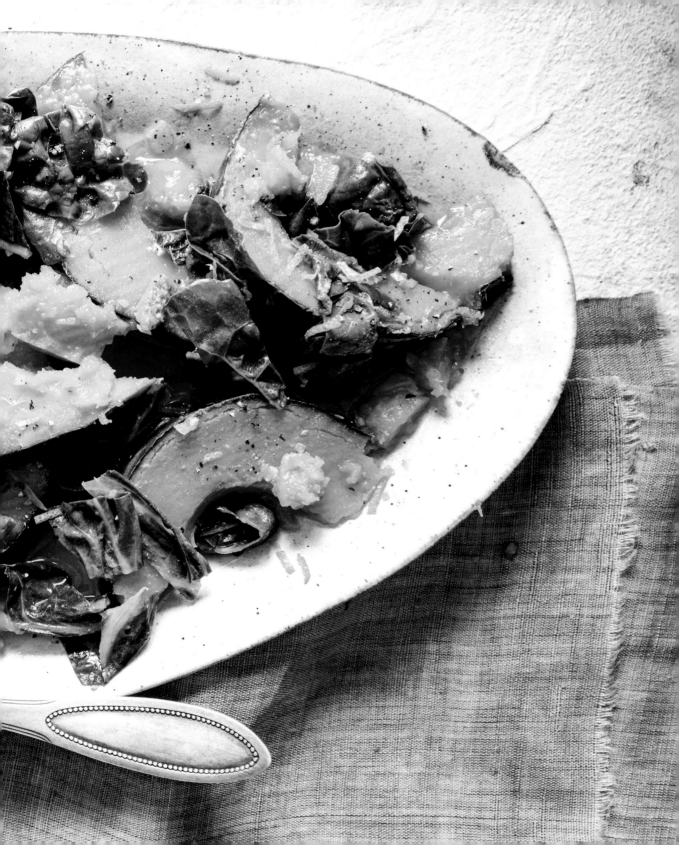

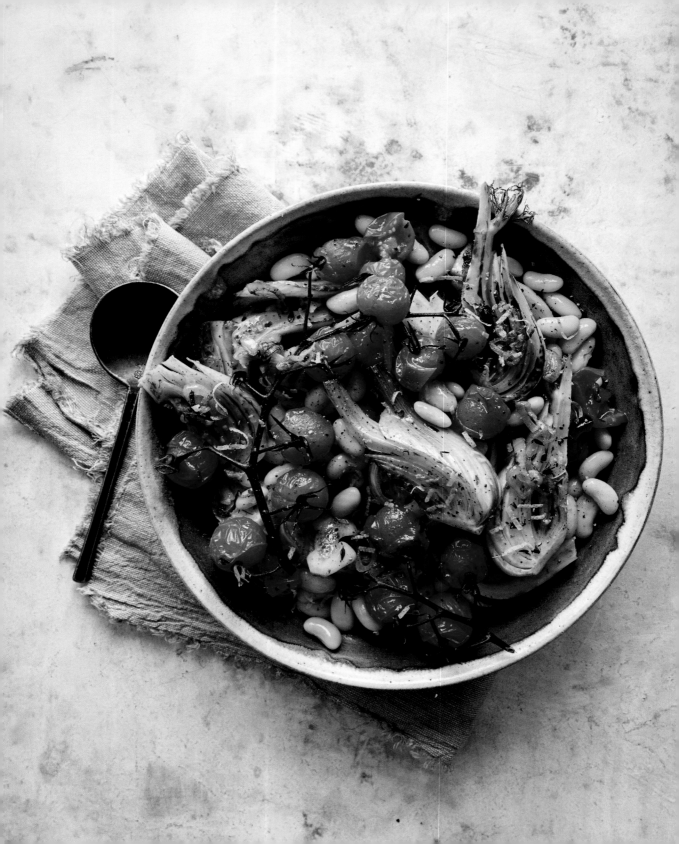

Roasted Fennel and Tomatoes

with White Beans

PREP TIME// 20 minutes

COOK TIME// 35 minutes

SERVES// 4

1 shallot, peeled and thinly sliced

2 large fennel bulbs, fronds removed and discarded, cut into 1-inch wedges

3 cups cherry tomatoes

4 sprigs fresh thyme

3 garlic cloves, crushed

2 tablespoons avocado oil

Sea salt and freshly ground black pepper to taste

1 (15-ounce) can cannellini beans, drained and rinsed

1 lemon, zested and juiced

This sheet pan recipe is inspired by a crazy delicious dish made by my aunt Susan. Because everything is prepared and cooked on baking sheets in the oven, there's minimal cookware to wash. Roasting fennel brings out a unique caramelization of the anise flavor. Pairing the fennel with cherry tomatoes is the perfect summer combination because the in-season tomatoes will be at their sweetest.

1 Preheat the oven to 425°F. Line two baking sheets with parchment paper.

2 In a large bowl, toss the shallot, fennel, tomatoes, thyme, and garlic with avocado oil. Spread out evenly between the prepared baking sheets without overcrowding and season with salt and pepper.

3 Roast for 30 to 35 minutes, flipping halfway through, until the tomatoes break down and the fennel is golden brown and very tender. Remove from the oven and add the beans during the last 5 to 8 minutes of cooking. Remove the thyme sprigs, stir in lemon zest and lemon juice, and serve.

Tomato Spanish Rice

with Caramelized Onions

PREP TIME// 10 minutes

COOK TIME// 1 hour

SERVES// 4

2 tablespoons avocado oil

2 medium yellow onions, thinly sliced

2 garlic cloves, minced

1 green bell pepper, cored, seeded, and diced

1 medium carrot, diced

Sea salt to taste

3 tablespoons tomato paste

1 teaspoon ground cumin

1 cup long-grain brown rice, rinsed

3½ to 4 cups water

1 cup frozen peas, thawed

¼ cup chopped fresh flat-leaf parsley, to garnish

¼ cup chopped fresh cilantro, to garnish

I've been making Spanish rice as a side dish for years. In this recipe, I caramelize the onions for a deep, rich flavor that pairs nicely with the tomato paste. I also use brown rice rather than white rice for added fiber, which helps keep me full longer since the brown rice takes longer to digest—good for times when I'm not in high-intensity training.

1 In a medium saucepan, heat the avocado oil over medium-high heat. Add the onions and cook for 10 minutes, stirring frequently, or until golden brown. Add the garlic, bell pepper, and carrot and cook another 3 to 4 minutes, until softened. Season with salt. Add the tomato paste and cumin, cooking an additional minute until the tomato paste is caramelized and the cumin is toasted and fragrant.

2 Add the rice and 3½ cups of the water. Bring to a boil, then reduce to a simmer, cover, and allow to cook for 40 to 45 minutes. Add an additional ½ cup water if the pan is dry but the rice needs to cook further. Fluff the rice with a fork, stir in the peas, and garnish with parsley and cilantro.

SERVING TIP: For a complete meal, add a fried egg and a quarter of an avocado to each plate!

Rinny and Tim O'Donnell's Smashed Potatoes

ATHLETE RECIPE: Originally from Australia and now residing in Boulder, Colorado, Mirinda O'Donnell, with more than fifty wins at major events throughout the world, is a threat at every race she enters. Her Ironman 70.3 World Championship title, three Ironman World titles, and seven podium finishes in the span of a decade mark her as one of the greatest triathletes of all time.

Timothy O'Donnell is an American long-course triathlete with more than fifty podium finishes, including more than twenty-five wins at major events throughout the world. Before dedicating his career to Ironman racing, Tim represented the navy with six consecutive wins at the Armed Forces National Championship and the United States with a win at the 2009 ITU Long Distance World Championship. At the 2019 Ironman World Championship in Kona, Hawaii, Timothy finished in second place. His sub-eight-hour performance was the fastest time ever recorded by an American at the World Championship.

"This potato smash has become a family favorite and one of our go-to side options. Super tasty, easy to prepare, and nutrient rich—plus, it's super filling, which is a huge priority when you are racking up the hours on long Ironman training weeks."

PREP TIME// 10 minutes
COOK TIME// 45 minutes
SERVES// 4

1 Preheat the oven to 425°F. Line a baking sheet with parchment paper.

2 Place the potatoes in a large pot and cover with cold, salted water. Bring to a boil, then reduce to a simmer and cook for 15 to 20 minutes, until tender. Drain and allow to cool.

3 On the prepared baking sheet, toss together the potatoes, olive oil, garlic, and thyme. Season with salt and pepper. Using the bottom of a drinking glass, press down on the potatoes to smash them flat. Bake for 20 to 25 minutes on the bottom rack, until the bottoms are golden brown and crispy.

4 Remove from the oven and sprinkle with flaky sea salt, if desired.

1 pound baby multicolored potatoes

¼ cup extra-virgin olive oil

2 garlic cloves, minced

1 teaspoon fresh thyme

Sea salt and freshly ground black pepper to taste

Flaky sea salt, to garnish (optional)

Aisha Praught-Leer's Jamaican Rice and Peas

ATHLETE RECIPE: Aisha Praught-Leer is a dual citizen of the United States and Jamaica and a two-time Olympian. She competes internationally for Jamaica, holding five national records and Jamaica's only global medals above 800 meters in the Commonwealth Games, gold in the 3,000-meter Steeplechase, and Pan Am Games silver in the 1,500 meter. She lives and trains in Boulder, Colorado, with Team Boss alongside some of the most accomplished and encouraging women in the world. Outside of running, she loves spending time with her husband and dog, reading books, being outside, and experimenting in the kitchen.

"Traditionally served on Sundays in Jamaica, rice and peas (beans) is a staple dish served in Jamaican households all over the world. I usually make it to fuel my Sunday long runs because it's full of healthy fats, protein, and carbs. I prefer white rice before long-run days because it's easier on my stomach. Since written recipes aren't the norm in my family, I learned how to make this dish at my sister's house in Ocho Rios and have adapted it to ingredients found easily in the States. I also use canned kidney beans to save time (sorry, fam)."

1 Pour the reserved bean liquid into a liquid measuring cup. Add enough water to total 1½ cups of liquid.

2 In a medium pot or Dutch oven, bring to a boil the bean liquid and water mixture, beans, onion, scallions, garlic, ginger, Scotch bonnet, allspice, and thyme. Season with salt and pepper and give a stir. Add the rice and coconut milk and stir again.

3 Once the pot returns to a gentle boil, reduce the heat to a simmer and cover, stirring occasionally. Allow to cook for 20 to 25 minutes, until all the liquid is absorbed. Remove the thyme sprigs and Scotch bonnet. Fluff the rice with a fork and serve.

PREP TIME// 10 minutes
COOK TIME// 30 minutes
SERVES// 4 to 6

1 (15-ounce) can no-salt-added kidney beans, drained and liquid reserved

1 medium onion (any color), diced

2 scallions or spring onions (white and green parts), sliced

3 garlic cloves, minced

1 (1-inch) piece of ginger, peeled and grated

1 Scotch bonnet or habanero pepper

8 allspice berries or ¼ teaspoon ground allspice

8 sprigs of fresh thyme

Sea salt and freshly ground black pepper to taste

2 cups long-grain white rice, rinsed

1 (13.5-ounce) can full-fat coconut milk

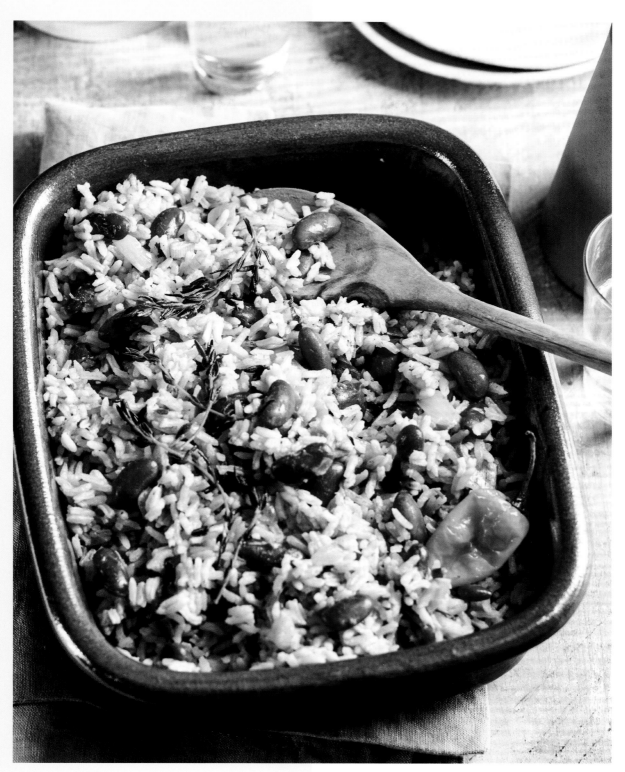

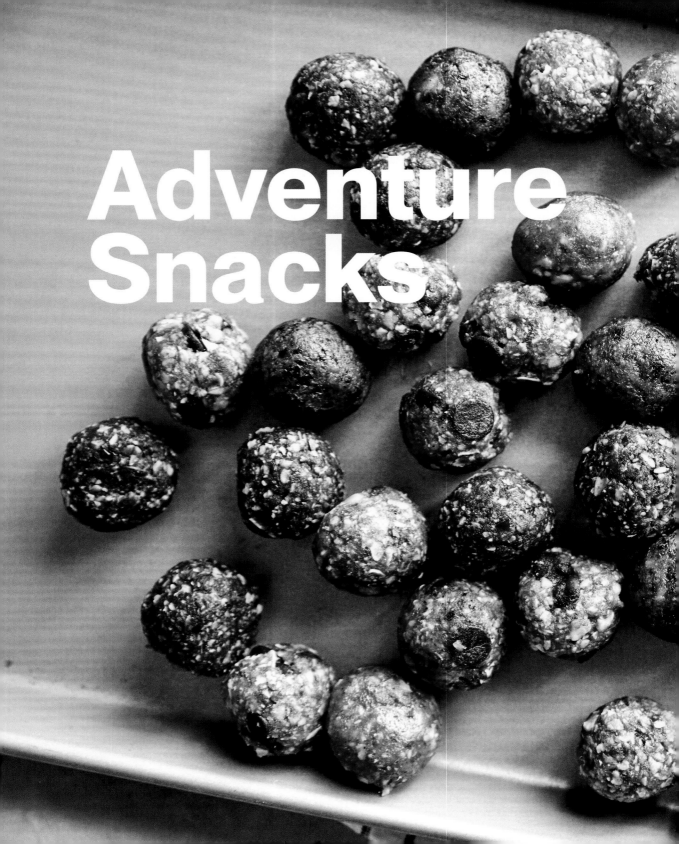

Adventure Snacks

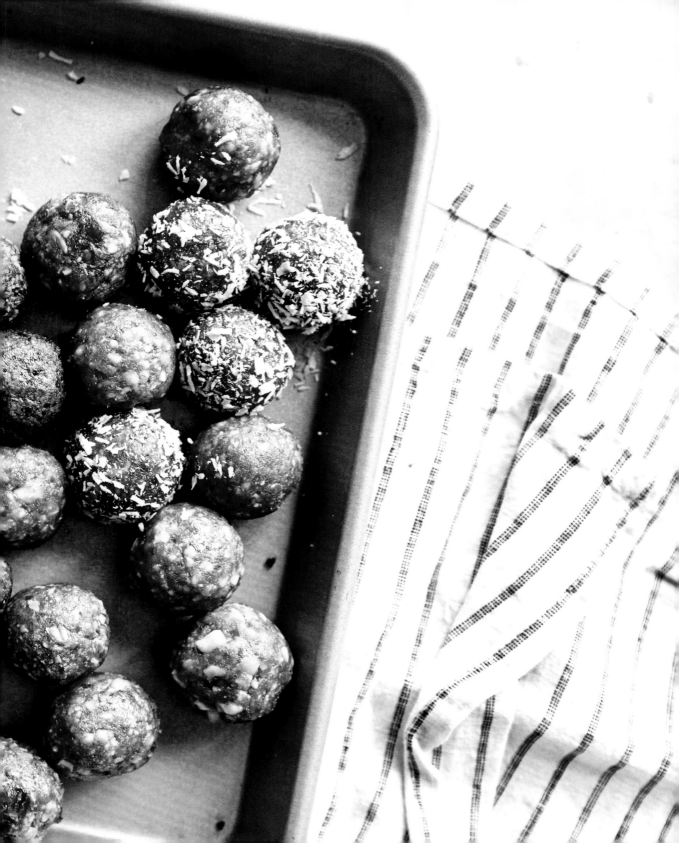

Athletes demand body fuel for training, but everyone can benefit from learning how to power their bodies to perform at the highest level, whether it's in fitness or everyday life. With my adventure snacks, I'm using the term *adventure* broadly. These snacks can be used to fuel all different activities, and they are also meant to be easily portable. So whether you have a long car or plane ride ahead of you or a bike ride, hike, or workout, swap these homemade snacks for your regular prepacked store-bought items. Using natural ingredients helps you control what you are eating for lasting all-day energy.

My personal favorites are the Peanut Butter Compost Cookies (page 188), which have a great texture and aren't too sweet. The Date Bites (pages 191–93) are what I'm most famous for, and I've included my six flavor variations for you to try. Since many of the snack recipes tend to be on the sweeter side, the Everything Bagel Trail Bar (page 201) provides a welcome savory twist.

Fueling Tip: Ever hit a wall while exercising? Known as bonking, this is when your energy completely plummets. There are several causes, but most commonly it's a result of total glycogen depletion from the muscles and liver. If you plan on exercising for 2 or more hours, it's important to fuel correctly to maintain your energy levels and avoid hitting that wall.

Long-Ride (Cycling) Tip: Aim to drink at least 1 bottle of fluid every hour. Depending on heat and intensity, alternate between electrolytes and water. A notable difference between running and riding is that when riding, the body is able to digest real food. This is because the action of running causes more physical stress on your GI system. If you plan to ride for more than 2 hours, be sure to think about fueling. The adventure snacks in this chapter offer some real-food fuel options for long rides! The recipes I have on repeat are the Miso Sweet Potato Rice Snacks (page 195) and the Peanut Butter Compost Cookies (page 188).

Long-Run Tip: A long run is typically considered 75 minutes or longer, and fueling is critical. As a general rule, aim to consume 100 calories every hour with a focus on simple carbohydrates, 30 to 60 grams. Remember, each person's body is different and will require a different fueling strategy.

Fueling Tip: For day-to-day nutritional goals, avoiding processed simple sugars is recommended. But during exercise, these sugars are exactly what the body needs. Simple sugars are stripped of most of their nutrients and therefore will take less energy for your body to digest.

Caffeine Tip while Running: Be sure when fueling to keep track of your caffeine intake. A good strategy is to consume caffeine later rather than earlier in a run. This helps keep your energy levels stable, so you don't feel an energy drain mid- or late run.

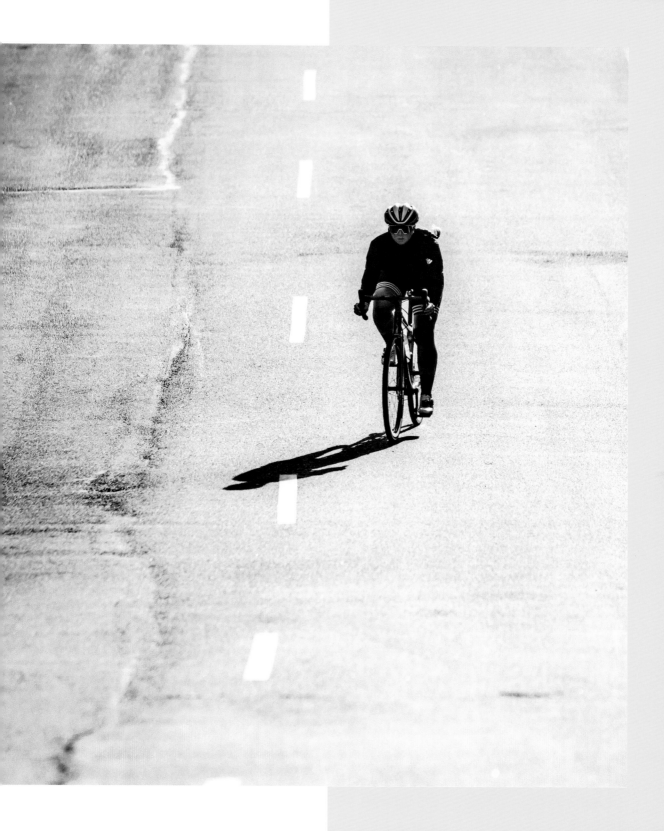

Fig and Oat Bars

PREP TIME// 20 minutes +
15 minutes soaking + overnight
refrigeration
COOK TIME// 50 minutes
MAKES// 15 bars

Coconut oil, for greasing

Filling

2 cups dried Turkish figs, halved

Hot water (115°F to 120°F), to
cover figs

1 orange, zested

2 to 3 tablespoons fresh orange juice

¼ teaspoon sea salt

Dough

2½ cups oat flour

2½ cups old-fashioned rolled oats

⅔ cup raw pecans, chopped

1 teaspoon ground cinnamon

1 tablespoon ground flaxseed

½ teaspoon sea salt

½ cup pure maple syrup

½ cup coconut oil, melted

3 large eggs, lightly beaten

½ cup unsweetened nut milk

1 teaspoon vanilla extract

These bars are inspired by a classic Fig Newton and adapted for the trail. The oats and pecans make a sturdy granola bar base that holds the jammy orange and fig center. These bars are also a great midafternoon treat with a coffee since they aren't too sweet and will keep you full until dinner.

1 Preheat the oven to 350°F. Grease an 11 × 7-inch baking dish with coconut oil and line with parchment paper, letting some overhang on the sides as handles.

2 **For the Filling:** In a small heatproof bowl, cover the figs with hot water and allow to soak for 15 minutes to soften. Drain the figs, reserving the liquid.

3 Transfer the figs to the bowl of a food processor fitted with the blade attachment. Add the orange zest, orange juice, and salt and puree until smooth. If the mixture is too thick, add some of the reserved soaking liquid, a tablespoon at a time, until a jam consistency forms. Set aside.

4 **For the Dough:** In a large bowl, whisk together the flour, oats, pecans, cinnamon, flaxseed, and salt.

5 In a medium bowl, combine the maple syrup, coconut oil, eggs, nut milk, and vanilla. Make a well in the dry ingredients and pour the wet ingredients inside. Mix gently until just combined.

6 Press half the dough into the bottom of the prepared baking dish. Spread the fig mixture on top. Crumble the remaining dough on top of the fig mixture and press down gently.

7 Bake for 40 to 50 minutes on the middle rack, until lightly browned. Allow to cool completely in the pan. Cover the bars and refrigerate overnight to allow the filling to set. Slice into 15 small bars and store in an airtight container in the refrigerator for up to 3 days.

TIP: Use your favorite dried fruit and nuts in this recipe. Dates also work really well!

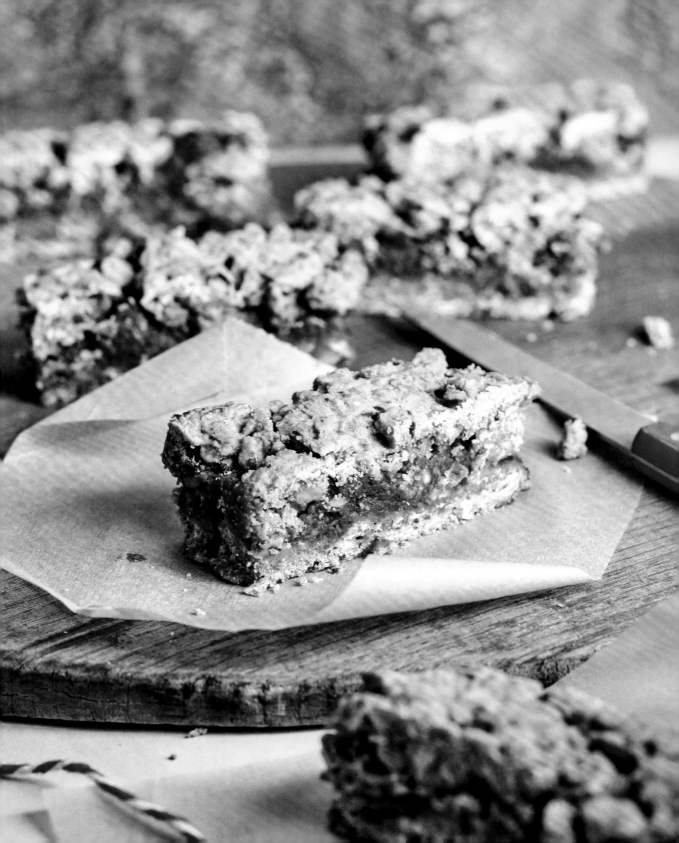

Coconut Matcha Fat Bites

PREP TIME// 20 minutes

MAKES// 16 bites

1 cup old-fashioned rolled oats

½ cup unsweetened coconut flakes, plus additional for rolling

¼ cup unsweetened natural almond butter

⅓ cup raw walnuts

2 tablespoons ground flaxseed

1 to 2 tablespoons matcha, plus additional for rolling

½ cup pitted Medjool dates, halved

½ teaspoon sea salt

3 to 4 tablespoons hot water (115°F to 120°F)

I'm a fan of matcha as an alternative form of caffeine. Because matcha has a slower release of caffeine than coffee, it lasts longer in your system and makes you less jittery. This recipe is designed as a bite-sized caffeine boost that can be eaten before, during, or after a workout. Note that a fat bite is different from an energy bite and is meant to keep you full longer. This is because fats are digested by the body more slowly than carbs. I find that fat bites are great to take on daily outings as well as on longer adventures.

1 In the bowl of a food processor fitted with the blade attachment, pulse the oats, coconut flakes, almond butter, walnuts, flaxseed, matcha, dates, and salt until just combined, adding hot water as necessary, until the dough forms a ball.

2 In a baking dish, mix together the additional coconut flakes and matcha. Roll the dough into 1½-inch balls and roll the balls in the coconut-matcha mixture. Store in an airtight container in the refrigerator for up to a few months.

TIPS: Hemp or chia seeds are a great protein addition to these fat bites.

If you are not a matcha fan, you can omit from this recipe, but if you still want the caffeine boost, then try subbing the same amount of maca powder.

Banana Peanut Oat Bars

PREP TIME// 10 minutes

COOK TIME// 28 minutes

MAKES// 12 bars

Coconut oil cooking spray,
for greasing

2 cups old-fashioned rolled oats

⅓ cup roasted unsalted peanuts

⅓ cup stevia-sweetened dark
chocolate chips (I like Lily's)

2 tablespoons ground flaxseed

½ teaspoon ground cinnamon

2 bananas, mashed (about 1 cup)

½ cup unsweetened natural creamy
peanut butter

1 large egg, lightly beaten

3 tablespoons pure maple syrup

2 teaspoons vanilla extract

½ teaspoon sea salt

Perfect to pack for a workout adventure or long outing, these taste like banana bread turned into an oat bar. Lots of peanut-y flavor with a hint of banana and cinnamon makes for a delicious afternoon snack. Peanuts are high in healthy fats as well as protein and fiber. They also contain potassium, B vitamins, and magnesium, which helps regulate fluid balance, energy levels, and blood sugar levels in the body.

1 Preheat the oven to 350°F. Grease an 8 × 8-inch baking dish with cooking spray and line with parchment paper, allowing the sides to overhang as handles.

2 Place the oats, peanuts, chocolate chips, flaxseed, and cinnamon in a medium bowl.

3 In a large bowl, whisk together the bananas, peanut butter, egg, maple syrup, vanilla, and salt until smooth.

4 Make a well in the oat mixture. Add the banana mixture to the well and mix until just combined. Press evenly into the prepared baking dish and smooth the top. Bake for 25 to 28 minutes, until golden brown and set.

5 Allow the bars to cool completely in the pan before slicing into 12 bars and serving. Store in an airtight container in the refrigerator for up to 4 days.

TIP: Feel free to use your favorite nuts and nut butter in these bars.

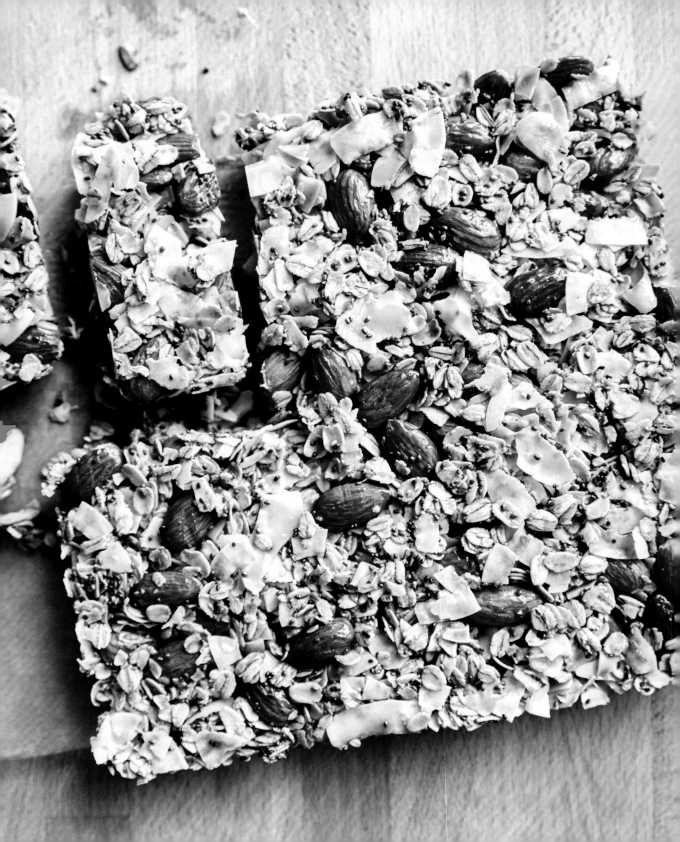

Chia Almond Coconut Bars

PREP TIME// 15 minutes

COOK TIME// 30 minutes

MAKES// 12 bars

1½ cups old-fashioned rolled oats

1 cup raw almonds

1 cup unsweetened coconut flakes

2 tablespoons chia seeds

¼ cup pure maple syrup

¼ teaspoon sea salt

3 large egg whites

Inspired by a store-bought granola bar, these bars have lots of crunch with a hint of sweetness. Coconut flakes are the prime ingredient for the texture in these bars and also provide a lot of health benefits. Coconut contains healthy fats, B vitamins, and manganese, which is needed for bone health and the breakdown of carbs. Coconut also happens to be a good source of iron and copper, which are both important for red blood cell formation.

1 Preheat the oven to 325°F. Line an 8 × 8-inch baking dish with parchment paper, letting the sides overhang as handles.

2 In a large bowl, combine the oats, almonds, coconut flakes, chia seeds, maple syrup, and salt.

3 In a small bowl, beat the egg whites using a fork until lightly frothy. Pour over the oat mixture and toss until lightly coated. Place into the prepared baking dish and press down to flatten with a rubber spatula. Bake for 25 to 30 minutes, until golden brown and set.

4 Allow to cool completely in the pan. Remove from the pan and slice into 12 bars. Store in an airtight container at room temperature for up to 4 days.

TIPS: I love adding a chocolate drizzle on top of these bars, either by mixing cocoa powder and coconut oil or by melting stevia-sweetened dark chocolate chips. But if you're taking these on an adventure, I recommend omitting the drizzle since it tends to be messy in your bag or pocket.

I always make these bars in advance and keep them in the freezer for up to 1 month for an easy homemade snack.

Peanut Butter Compost Cookies

PREP TIME// 15 minutes

COOK TIME// 12 minutes

MAKES// 16 cookies

1 cup unsweetened natural creamy peanut butter

½ cup pure maple syrup

¼ cup coconut oil, melted

2 large eggs, at room temperature, lightly beaten

2 teaspoons vanilla extract

1 teaspoon sea salt

1½ cups almond flour

1 teaspoon baking soda

1 teaspoon baking powder

1 cup old-fashioned rolled oats

½ cup cacao nibs

½ cup dried raisins

½ cup pecans, chopped

These cookies hold up really well during a long bike ride, aren't too sweet to eat in the middle of a workout, and are also a great anytime dessert! I use maple syrup as a natural sweetener for several of my desserts and adventure snacks in addition to dates or fruit. Maple syrup has some minerals and antioxidants, like manganese, as well as a slightly lower glycemic index than regular sugar. Be sure you are buying pure maple syrup when you go to the store and not artificially sweetened maple-flavored syrup.

1 Preheat the oven to 350°F. Line two baking sheets with parchment paper.

2 In a large bowl, stir together the peanut butter, maple syrup, and coconut oil until smooth. Add the eggs, one at a time, and mix until just incorporated. Stir in the vanilla and salt.

3 In a medium bowl, whisk together the salt, flour, baking soda, and baking powder. Fold the dry ingredients into the nut butter mixture and add the oats, cacao nibs, raisins, and pecans.

4   Using a ¼-cup measure, scoop the cookie dough onto the prepared baking sheets. Press lightly with your fingers to flatten the top of the cookies. Bake for 10 to 12 minutes, until golden and just set. Allow to cool on the pan completely and serve.

TIP: Use any dried fruit or nut butter you desire in this recipe.

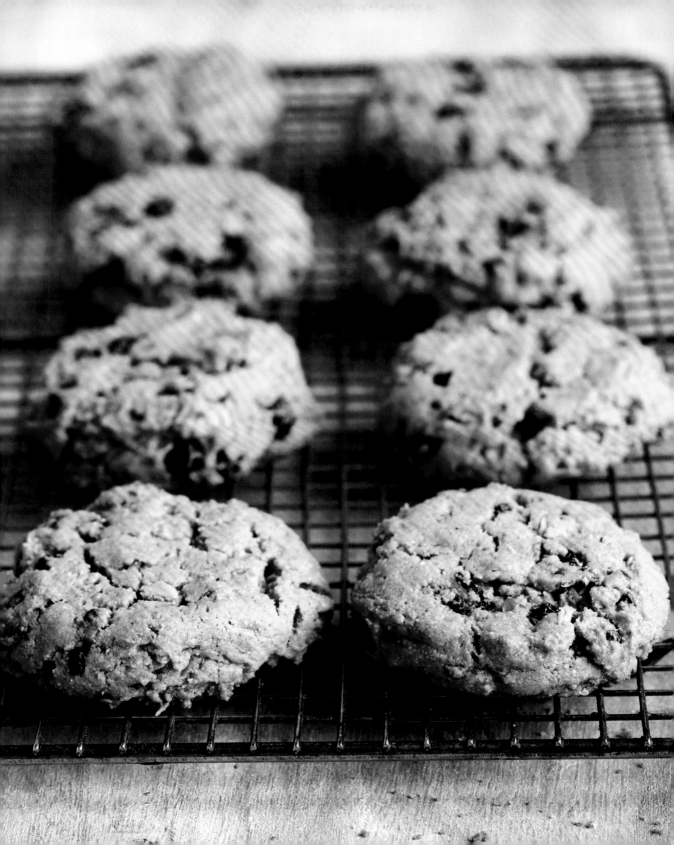

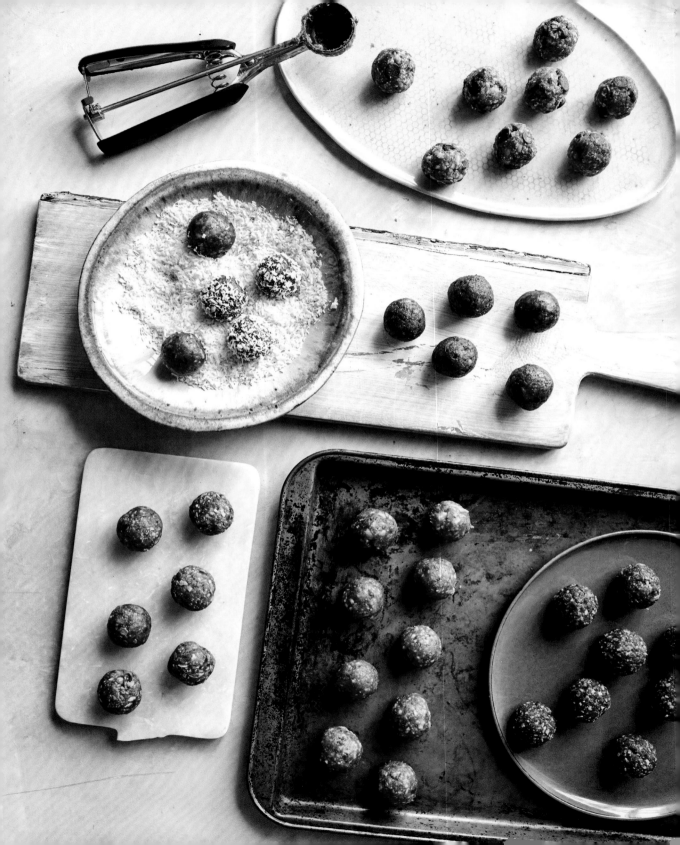

Date Bites
Six Ways

These date bites were the start to my career when I was seventeen. I was interested in learning more about natural health foods and started selling date bites as a small business in high school. In college, I began my food blog, *Running on Veggies,* and shared this date bites recipe. They are still one of my most popular workout snacks. With six awesome flavors and endless more combinations, these date bites are great for a pre- or post-workout treat. They are best in cold-weather seasons, so they don't melt in your pocket.

Original

PREP TIME// 20 minutes + 10 minutes soaking

MAKES// 20 bites

2 cups pitted Medjool dates, halved

Hot water (115°F to 120°F), to cover dates

2 cups raw whole nuts of choice, or 1 cup raw whole nuts + 1 cup old-fashioned rolled oats

3 tablespoons unsweetened natural nut butter of choice

1 tablespoon vanilla extract

2 teaspoons ground cinnamon

½ teaspoon sea salt

Optional Add-Ins

1 to 2 tablespoons cacao powder

Chia seeds

Flaxseeds

Protein powder

1 In a small heatproof bowl, cover the dates with hot water and allow to soak for 10 minutes to soften. Drain and discard the liquid.

2 In the bowl of a food processor fitted with the blade attachment, pulse the nuts until roughly chopped. Add the softened dates, nut butter, vanilla, cinnamon, salt, and add-ins (if using) and pulse until a dough forms. Roll the mixture into 1½-inch balls and refrigerate in an airtight container until ready to serve.

TIP: This is a great base recipe for all your unique date ball flavor combinations. These can be stored in an airtight container in the refrigerator for up to 2 weeks or in the freezer for up to 2 months.

Coffee

PREP TIME// 20 minutes + 10 minutes soaking

MAKES// 20 bites

2 cups pitted Medjool dates, halved

Hot water (115°F to 120°F), to cover dates

2 cups raw walnuts

¼ cup whole roasted coffee beans

1 tablespoon pure vanilla extract

2 teaspoons ground cinnamon

½ teaspoon sea salt

1 In a small heatproof bowl, cover the dates with hot water and allow to soak for 10 minutes to soften. Drain and discard the liquid.

2 In the bowl of a food processor fitted with the blade attachment, pulse the walnuts and coffee beans until roughly chopped. Add the softened dates, vanilla, cinnamon, and salt and pulse until a dough forms. Roll the mixture into 1½-inch balls and refrigerate in an airtight container until ready to serve.

Peanut Butter Chocolate

PREP TIME// 20 minutes + 10 minutes soaking

MAKES// 20 bites

2 cups pitted Medjool dates, halved

Hot water (115°F to 120°F), to cover dates

1 cup unsalted roasted peanuts

1 cup old-fashioned rolled oats

3 tablespoons unsweetened natural creamy peanut butter

2 tablespoons unsweetened cocoa powder

1 tablespoon vanilla extract

½ teaspoon sea salt

1 to 2 tablespoons cold water, if needed

1   In a small heatproof bowl, cover the dates with hot water and allow to soak for 10 minutes to soften. Drain and discard the liquid.

2   In the bowl of a food processor fitted with the blade attachment, pulse the peanuts until roughly chopped. Add the softened dates, oats, peanut butter, cocoa powder, vanilla, and salt and pulse until a dough forms. Add cold water to loosen the dough if needed. Roll the mixture into 1½-inch balls and refrigerate in an airtight container until ready to serve.

Cookie Dough

PREP TIME// 20 minutes + 10 minutes soaking

MAKES// 20 bites

2 cups pitted Medjool dates, halved

Hot water (115°F to 120°F), to cover dates

1 cup raw almonds

1 cup old-fashioned rolled oats

3 tablespoons unsweetened natural almond butter

1 tablespoon vanilla extract

½ teaspoon sea salt

½ cup stevia-sweetened dark chocolate chips (I like Lily's)

1   In a small heatproof bowl, cover the dates with hot water and allow to soak for 10 minutes to soften. Drain and discard the liquid.

2   In the bowl of a food processor fitted with the blade attachment, pulse the almonds until roughly chopped. Add the softened dates, oats, almond butter, vanilla, and salt and pulse until a dough forms. Transfer to a large bowl and stir in the chocolate chips. Roll into 1½-inch balls and refrigerate in an airtight container until ready to serve.

Pecan Pie

PREP TIME// 20 minutes + 10 minutes soaking

MAKES// 20 bites

2 cups pitted Medjool dates, halved

Hot water (115°F to 120°F), to cover dates

2 cups raw pecans

3 tablespoons unsweetened natural almond butter

1 tablespoon vanilla extract

½ teaspoon ground cinnamon

Pinch of freshly grated nutmeg

½ teaspoon sea salt

1 cup unsweetened shredded coconut, for rolling

1 In a small heatproof bowl, cover the dates with hot water and allow to soak for 10 minutes to soften. Drain and discard the liquid.

2 In the bowl of a food processor fitted with the blade attachment, pulse the pecans until roughly ground. Add the softened dates, almond butter, vanilla, cinnamon, nutmeg, and salt and pulse until a dough forms.

3 Place the shredded coconut in a shallow bowl or baking dish. Roll the date bites into 1½-inch balls, then roll in the coconut to lightly coat. Refrigerate in an airtight container until ready to serve.

PB&J

PREP TIME// 20 minutes + 10 minutes soaking

MAKES// 20 bites

2 cups pitted Medjool dates, halved

Hot water (115°F to 120°F), to cover dates

1 cup unsalted roasted peanuts

1 cup old-fashioned rolled oats

3 tablespoons unsweetened natural creamy peanut butter

2 to 3 tablespoons fruit-sweetened raspberry jam

1 tablespoon vanilla extract

½ teaspoon sea salt

1 In a small heatproof bowl, cover the dates with hot water and allow to soak for 10 minutes to soften. Drain and discard the liquid.

2 In the bowl of a food processor fitted with the blade attachment, pulse the peanuts until roughly chopped. Add the softened dates, oats, peanut butter, jam, vanilla, and salt and pulse until a dough forms. Roll the mixture into 1½-inch balls and refrigerate in an airtight container until ready to serve.

Nut Cluster Cookies

PREP TIME// 10 minutes

COOK TIME// 20 minutes

MAKES// 20 cookies

3 tablespoons ground flaxseed

6 tablespoons water

1 cup roasted unsalted almonds, chopped

1 cup raw walnuts, chopped

1 cup raw pecans, chopped

½ cup old-fashioned rolled oats

½ cup stevia-sweetened dark chocolate chips (I like Lily's)

¼ cup sesame seeds

½ cup pure maple syrup

½ teaspoon vanilla extract

½ teaspoon sea salt

My mom and I came up with this recipe and they're a delicious nutty snack. The cookies are full of protein and vitamins from the nuts and sesame seeds, and they have a hint of sweetness from the maple. We love taking them on the go for a midday protein bite.

1 Preheat the oven to 350°F. Line a baking sheet with parchment paper.

2 In a medium bowl, mix together the flaxseed and water and allow to thicken for 5 minutes.

3 In a large bowl, combine the almonds, walnuts, pecans, oats, chocolate chips, and sesame seeds.

4 Add the maple syrup, vanilla, and salt to the thickened flax mixture and whisk to combine. Pour over the nut mixture and mix to combine.

5 Scoop the dough using a cookie scoop (or a little less than ¼ cup) onto the prepared baking sheet about 1 inch apart. Press down lightly to flatten the tops with your fingers (it's okay if they look like they're falling apart). Bake for 15 to 20 minutes, until golden and set. Allow to cool completely on the tray before serving. Store in an airtight container in the freezer for up to 4 days.

TIP: This recipe uses a vegan flax egg as the binder instead of regular eggs. A flax egg is 1 tablespoon ground flaxseed mixed with 2 tablespoons water in a bowl. Allow the mixture to thicken for 5 minutes and then use in your recipe. If you prefer to use eggs in this recipe, use 2 large eggs, lightly beaten, or 3 large egg whites.

Miso Sweet Potato Rice Snacks

PREP TIME// 10 minutes

COOK TIME// 30 minutes

MAKES// about 16 snacks

½ cup sushi rice

1 tablespoon toasted sesame oil

1 cup sweet potato, peeled and diced small

1 to 2 tablespoons water, plus additional if needed

2 teaspoons white or yellow miso paste

1 tablespoon liquid aminos (I like Bragg)

3 tablespoons fresh lemon juice

¼ cup raw sesame seeds

Sea salt to taste

2 to 3 sheets nori seaweed (7 by 8 inches each)

Inspired by sushi, these rice snacks are often used by cyclists since they are the perfect bite to pop into your pocket for a long endurance bike ride. The white sushi rice is higher in starch and sugar than regular white rice, which helps replenish the carbohydrates that your body quickly uses up during high-intensity workouts. Plus, the higher starch levels in the rice help hold this snack together nicely along with the seaweed wrapper. Seaweed is a great source of natural minerals and also provides electrolytes, which are essential in high-intensity workouts. The salty sweet flavors in this rice snack are so cravable during a strenuous workout.

1 Cook the sushi rice according to the package instructions. Allow to cool completely.

2 In a medium heavy-bottomed sauté pan or saucepan, heat the sesame oil over medium-low heat. Add the sweet potato and cook for 5 to 6 minutes, until tender. Add the water halfway through cooking to prevent the potato from burning. Add more water by the tablespoon if needed.

3 In a small bowl, whisk together the miso paste, liquid aminos, and lemon juice. Add to the pan during the last minute of cooking and toss to combine. Set aside and allow to cool completely.

4 In a large bowl, combine the cooled rice, sweet potato, and sesame seeds. Season with salt.

5 Cut the nori seaweed sheets in half lengthwise (about 4 x 3½ inches). Place 3 tablespoons of the rice mixture in one corner of one strip of nori. Form the rice mixture into a triangle shape. Fold the triangle diagonally to wrap the rice mixture completely in nori. Once you get to the end of the piece of nori, wet the end with water, and press to seal. Repeat with remaining rice and nori. Store in an airtight container in the refrigerator for up to 4 days.

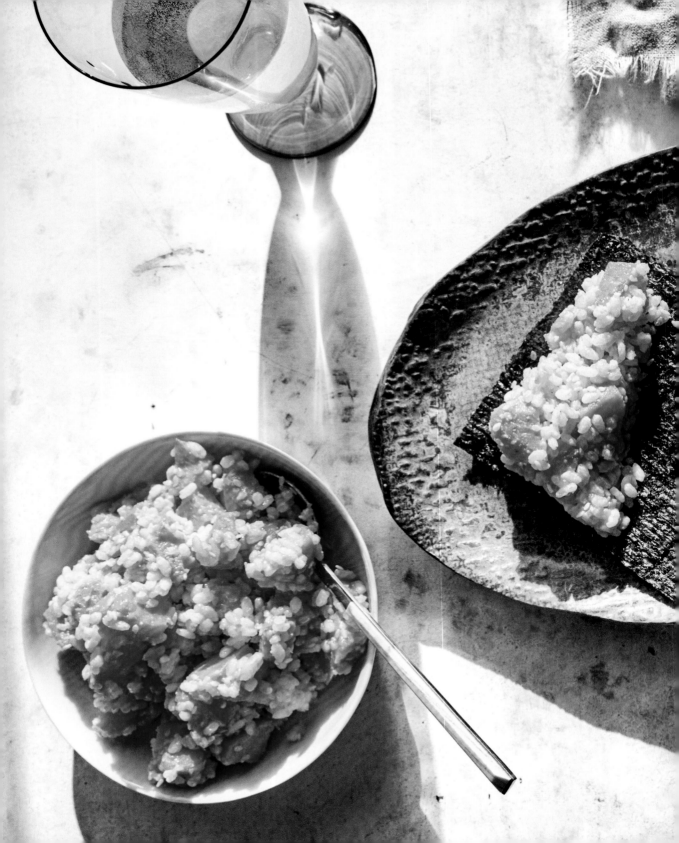

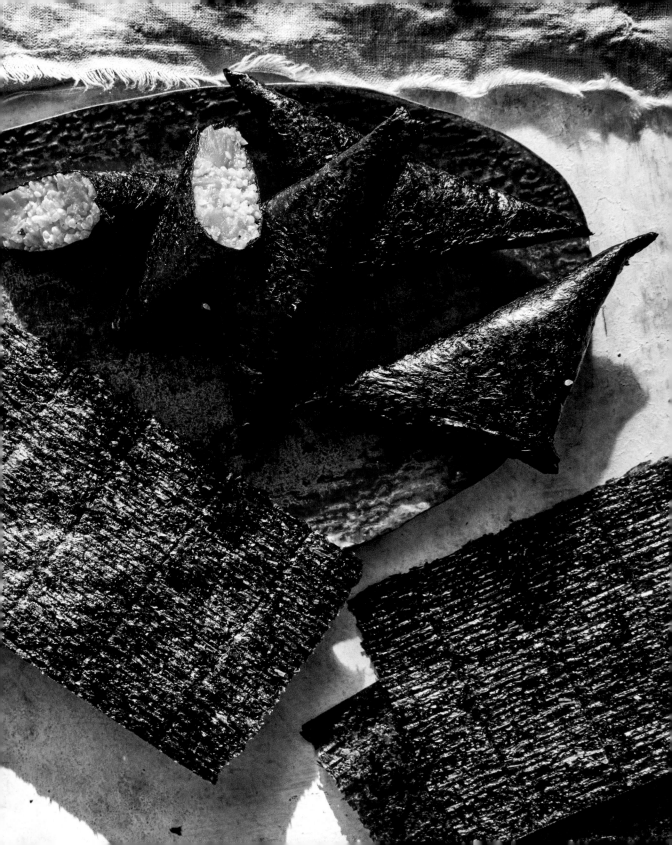

Spiced Nuts Trail Mix

PREP TIME// 10 minutes

COOK TIME// 18 minutes

MAKES// 5 cups

2 tablespoons avocado oil

2 tablespoons pure maple syrup

1 tablespoon dried thyme

1 teaspoon dried rosemary

Pinch of ground cinnamon

Pinch of cayenne pepper

1 teaspoon sea salt

1 cup raw walnuts

1 cup raw almonds

1 cup raw pecans

1 cup raw sunflower seeds

½ cup dried raisins

½ cup dried apricots, chopped

During the holiday season, this trail mix is a tasty treat I love gifting to friends and family. I either make the mix in full and bag it up or I make a trail mix kit with the dry ingredients in a mason jar and attach a recipe tag. It's the perfect afternoon snack and the perfect gift.

1 Preheat the oven to 350°F. Line a baking sheet with parchment paper.

2 In a small bowl, whisk together the avocado oil, maple syrup, thyme, rosemary, cinnamon, cayenne, and salt.

3 In a large bowl, combine the walnuts, almonds, and pecans. Pour the oil-syrup mixture over the nuts and toss evenly to coat. Spread the nuts into one layer on the prepared baking sheet. Roast for 15 to 18 minutes, flipping halfway through, until golden and fragrant. Remove from the oven and allow to cool almost completely.

4 Sprinkle the sunflower seeds, raisins, and apricots over the warm nuts and toss to combine. Store in an airtight container for up to 2 weeks.

TIP: Feel free to customize this recipe with your favorite nuts, spices, and dried fruits. If you want to keep this trail mix for longer than 2 weeks, I find it best to store in the freezer in an airtight container for up to 1 month.

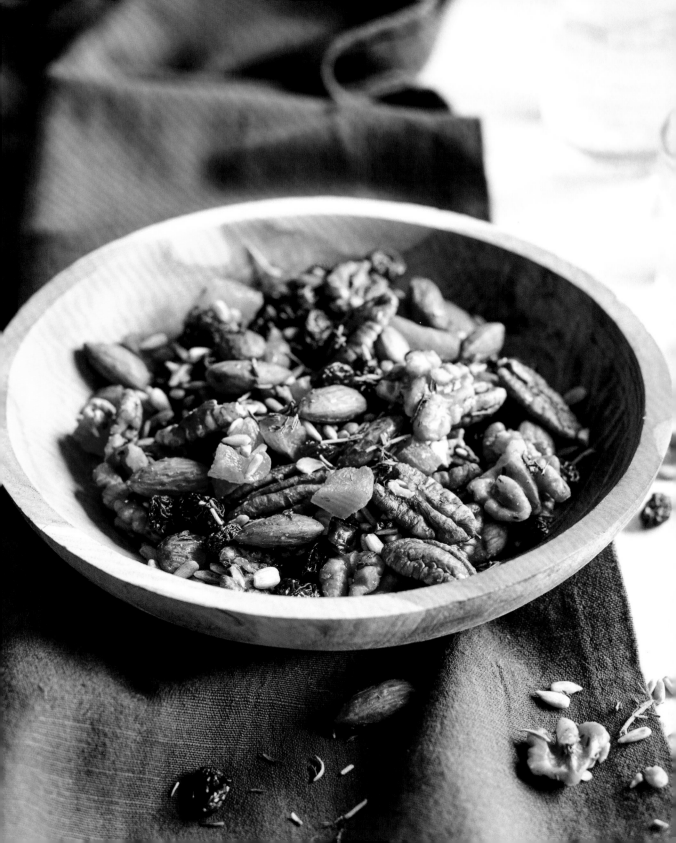

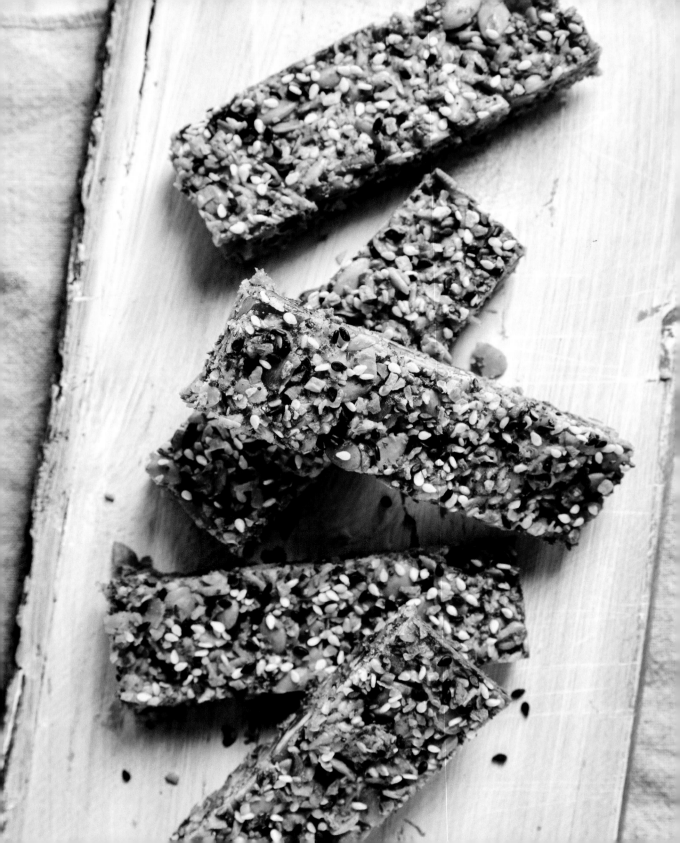

Everything Bagel Trail Bar

PREP TIME// 5 minutes +
20 minutes resting
COOK TIME// 1 hour 10 minutes
MAKES// 16 bars

1 cup old-fashioned rolled oats

½ cup raw pumpkin seeds

½ cup raw pecans, chopped

¼ cup ground flaxseed

2 tablespoons raw sesame seeds

2 tablespoons chia seeds

2 tablespoons Everything Bagel seasoning

½ teaspoon sea salt

2 tablespoons coconut oil, melted

2 tablespoons pure maple syrup

½ cup warm water

1 large egg, room temperature and lightly beaten

Being from New York City, I've always loved Everything Bagel seasoning. The combination of flavors is nutty and garlicky with a hint of onion and also pairs well with a touch of sweetness. Since there are so many sweet trail bars out there, I wanted to create a more savory bar and found that Everything Bagel spice was the perfect fit. These bars are an addicting sweet-and-salty snack great for any outing.

1 Preheat the oven to 300°F. Line an 8 × 8-inch baking dish with parchment paper, letting the sides overhang as handles.

2 In a large bowl, combine the oats, pumpkin seeds, pecans, flaxseed, sesame seeds, chia seeds, 1 tablespoon of the Everything Bagel seasoning, and salt.

3 In a small bowl, whisk together the coconut oil and maple syrup. Pour the oil-syrup mixture over the oat mixture and toss until evenly coated. Add the water and stir to combine. Allow to rest for 15 to 20 minutes, until the mixture thickens.

4 Once thickened, add the egg and toss to evenly coat. Scrape the mixture into the prepared baking dish and spread until smooth, pressing down with a rubber spatula. Sprinkle with the remaining 1 tablespoon Everything Bagel seasoning. Bake for 1 hour to 1 hour 10 minutes, until golden brown and set. Remove from the oven and allow to cool almost completely in the pan. Cut into bars and serve. Store in an airtight container for up to 3 days or in the freezer for 1 month.

Ian Boswell's Ginger Spice Cookies

ATHLETE RECIPE: Ian Boswell is a retired professional road cyclist who traveled the world and lived abroad for fifteen years during his professional career. Currently, he lives in Vermont with his wife on an old dairy farm and homestead. They enjoy keeping vegetable gardens, an apple orchard, chickens, and foraging seasonally.

"My wife and I love spending time together experimenting in the kitchen, and that's how these spice cookies were born. With so many hours and calories spent on the road, I'm always looking for something nutritious, homemade, and appetizing. I take these spice cookies on long bike rides for a quick snack when I'm in need of something sweet. The warm flavors satisfy my cravings and keep me pushing on my bike. Plus, these cookies have ginger for anti-inflammation as well as molasses, which is a good source of iron, making them the perfect mid-workout bite."

1 Preheat the oven to 375°F. Line two baking sheets with parchment paper.

2 For the Optional Sugar Topping: In a shallow bowl, combine the coconut sugar and cinnamon and set aside.

3 For the Cookies: In a medium bowl, whisk together the coconut oil, maple syrup, egg, molasses, and fresh ginger until smooth.

4 In a large bowl, whisk together the oat flour, almond flour, baking powder, cinnamon, ground ginger, nutmeg, and salt. Make a well in the dry ingredients and add the wet ingredients into the center of the well. Fold gently until just combined.

5 Using a cookie scoop or a tablespoon measure, scoop the dough onto the prepared baking sheets (each cookie is about 1½ tablespoons). Sprinkle the cookies with the sugar topping, if using, and gently press to flatten the cookie dough.

6 Bake for 10 to 12 minutes, until golden brown. Allow to cool completely on the pan before serving. Leftovers can be stored in an airtight container at room temperature for up to 3 days.

TIP: Molasses offers a lot of rich flavor in baked goods as well as health benefits. It's high in minerals, iron, calcium, potassium, and magnesium, which are beneficial to bone and blood health and reduce post-workout cramping.

PREP TIME// 15 minutes
COOK TIME// 12 minutes
MAKES// 18 cookies

Optional Sugar Topping

2 tablespoons coconut sugar

½ teaspoon ground cinnamon

Cookies

⅓ cup coconut oil, room temperature

⅓ cup pure maple syrup

1 large egg, room temperature

3 tablespoons molasses

1 teaspoon freshly grated ginger

1⅔ cups oat flour

1 cup almond flour

¾ teaspoon baking powder

1 teaspoon ground cinnamon

½ teaspoon ground ginger

¼ teaspoon ground nutmeg

¼ teaspoon sea salt

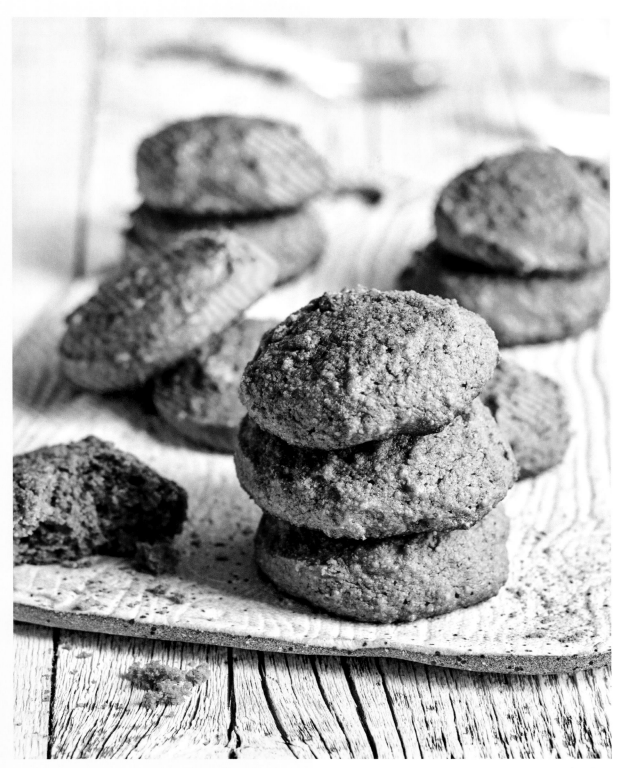

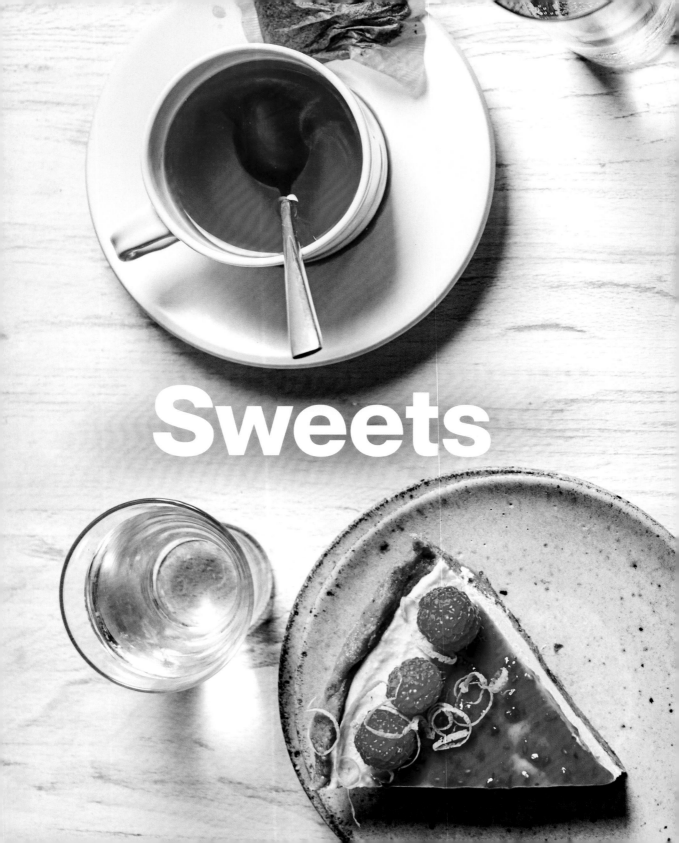

Sweets

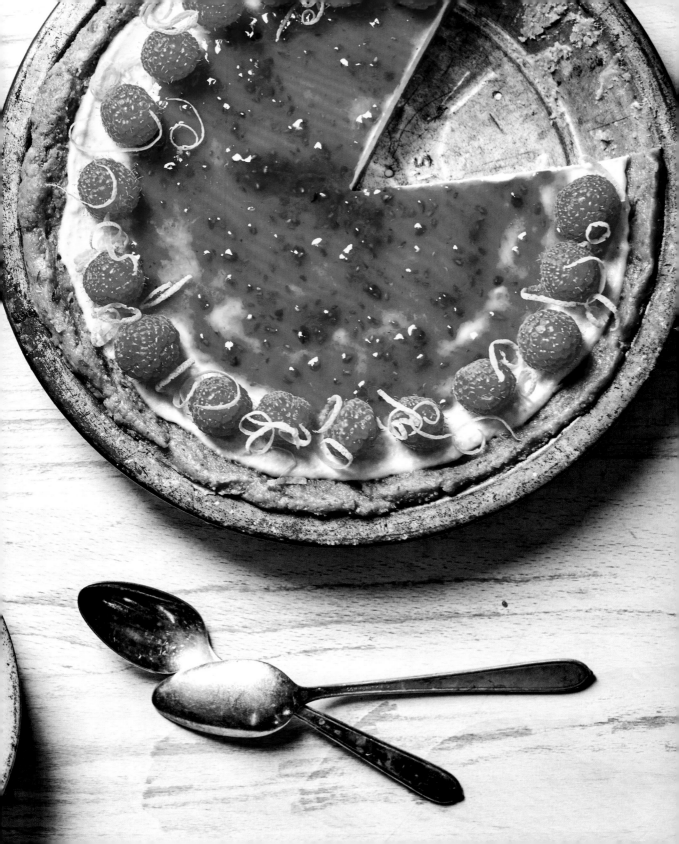

Whenever someone is hosting a dinner party, I'm always the first to offer to bring dessert! I love making sweets and coming up with vegan plant-based treats. What's different about my approach to making desserts is that I use natural sweeteners, like maple syrup, dates, and coconut sugar, because they have a lower glycemic index than other sweeteners typically found in desserts. Using these sweeteners allows all my favorite treats to be health focused without sacrificing taste, something I believe is so important! When it comes to flour in desserts, I also like to stick to almond and oat flours since they are packed with fiber and nutrients. They also are finely ground and light, creating a fluffy baked texture that is so delicious. For a sweet bite any time of day, try the Cinnamon Crumb Coffee Cake (page 213). If you are a cookie lover, the Chocolate Chip Oat Cookies (page 217) are so addictive. And the Double-Chocolate Cake with Chocolate Ganache (page 211) has become a birthday staple with my friends and family.

Flourless Fudgy Black Bean Brownies

PREP TIME// 15 minutes +
15 minutes soaking

COOK TIME// 30 minutes

MAKES// 8 brownies

Coconut oil cooking spray, for greasing

1 cup pitted Medjool dates, halved

Hot water (115°F to 120°F), to cover dates

1 (15-ounce) can black beans, drained and rinsed

2 large eggs

⅔ cup unsweetened cocoa powder

½ cup unsweetened applesauce

¼ cup pure maple syrup

2 teaspoons vanilla extract

½ teaspoon instant espresso (optional)

½ teaspoon baking soda

½ teaspoon baking powder

½ teaspoon sea salt

¾ cup stevia-sweetened dark chocolate chips (I like Lily's)

The ultimate melt-in-your-mouth brownies! They are so fudgy and chocolatey and hard to resist that you'd never know they are also gluten-free. It's amazing to think that black beans, which provide both fiber and potassium, are the hidden plant-based ingredient found in this decadent dessert!

1 Preheat the oven to 350°F. Line an 8 × 8-inch baking dish with parchment paper, allowing it to overhang for handles, and grease with cooking spray.

2 In a small heatproof bowl, cover the dates with hot water and allow to soak for 15 minutes to soften. Drain and discard the liquid.

3 Transfer the softened dates to the bowl of a food processor fitted with the blade attachment and add the black beans, eggs, cocoa powder, applesauce, maple syrup, vanilla, espresso (if using), baking soda, baking powder, and salt. Blend until smooth. Transfer the mixture to a large bowl and gently fold in ½ cup of the chocolate chips.

4 Smooth the batter evenly into the prepared baking dish and sprinkle with the remaining ¼ cup chocolate chips. Bake on the middle rack for 25 to 30 minutes, until the edges and top look set. Remove from the oven and allow to cool for 1 hour. Remove from the baking dish, slice, and serve. Store in an airtight container at room temperature for up to 4 days.

TIP: Adding instant espresso doesn't add coffee flavor to this dessert like you might think. The espresso actually helps bring out the richness and deep flavors of the cocoa powder, making this brownie a chocolate lover's dream.

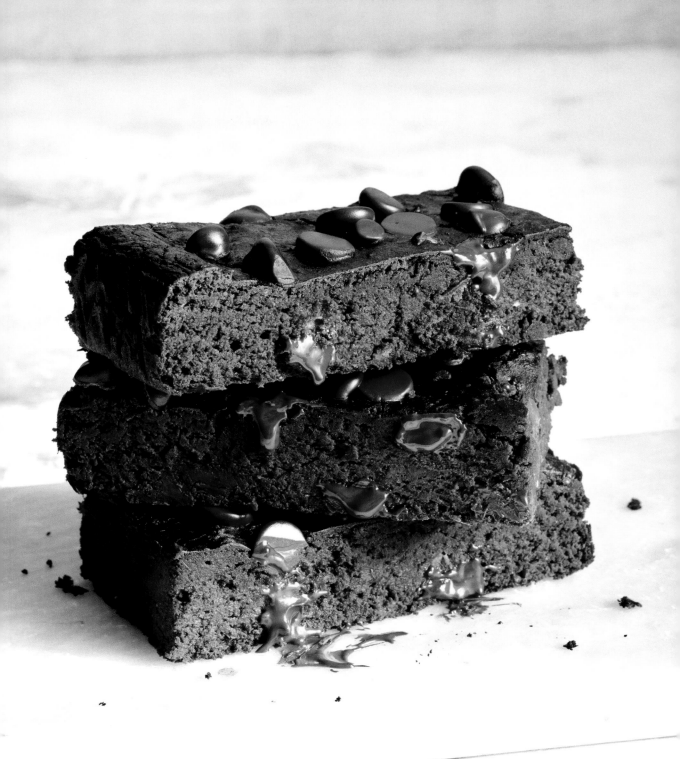

Nutty Tahini Fudge

PREP TIME// 10 minutes +
2 hours freezing

MAKES// 16 squares

2 cups tahini, well stirred

½ cup coconut oil, melted

⅓ cup pure maple syrup

1 tablespoon vanilla extract

⅓ cup toasted pecans, chopped

1 tablespoon black sesame seeds, to garnish (optional)

Flaky sea salt, to garnish

Tahini is a paste made from sesame seeds that has a delicious nutty flavor and is used in salad dressings, sauces, baked goods, and in this case, an elegant fudge recipe. I first developed this recipe for an athlete so they could add nutrients into a bite-size dessert. Tahini has so many health benefits: it contains several healthy fats and is a good source of calcium for bone health.

1 Line an 8 × 8-inch baking dish with parchment paper, allowing the paper to hang over the sides.

2 In a large bowl, whisk together the tahini, coconut oil, maple syrup, and vanilla until smooth. Fold in the pecans, then scrape the mixture into the prepared baking dish, smoothing the top. Garnish with the sesame seeds (if using) and a sprinkle of flaky sea salt.

3 Place in the freezer and allow to chill for 2 hours, or until firm. Remove from the freezer, slice into small squares, and serve. Store in an airtight container in the freezer for up to 1 month.

Double-Chocolate Cake
with Chocolate Ganache

PREP TIME// 15 minutes

COOK TIME// 45 minutes

MAKES// one 9-inch cake

Double-Chocolate Cake

Coconut oil cooking spray, for greasing

1½ cups oat flour

¾ cup almond flour

¾ cup unsweetened cocoa powder

1 teaspoon baking soda

1 teaspoon espresso powder

1 teaspoon sea salt

2 large eggs, lightly beaten

1 cup coconut sugar

¾ cup unsweetened nut milk

½ cup coconut oil, melted

2 teaspoons vanilla extract

1 tablespoon apple cider vinegar

¾ cup boiling water

Chocolate Ganache

1 cup stevia-sweetened dark chocolate chips (I like Lily's)

⅓ cup unsweetened nut milk

My family and friends always request this double-chocolate cake for birthdays. It was originally inspired by the classic chocolate box cakes that I made growing up. Using oat and almond flour makes this cake gluten-free and keeps the base light and fluffy. The decadent chocolate ganache is the perfect finish that adds even more rich chocolate flavor to every bite.

1 **For the Double-Chocolate Cake:** Preheat the oven to 350°F. Grease a 9-inch round cake pan with cooking spray and line with parchment paper.

2 In a large bowl, whisk together the oat flour, almond flour, cocoa powder, baking soda, espresso powder, and salt.

3 In a medium bowl, whisk together the eggs, coconut sugar, nut milk, coconut oil, vanilla, and vinegar.

4 Make a well in the dry ingredients and pour half the wet ingredients into the center of the well. Fold gently to combine. Slowly add the boiling water while stirring to avoid cooking the eggs. Add the remaining wet ingredient mixture and mix until just combined.

5 Place the batter into the prepared cake pan and smooth the top. Bake on the middle rack for 40 to 45 minutes, until an inserted toothpick comes out clean. Remove from the oven and allow to cool completely in the pan.

6 Once completely cooled, remove from the pan to a plate with a lip and discard the parchment.

7 **For the Chocolate Ganache:** Place the chocolate chips in a medium heatproof bowl. In a small saucepan, bring the nut milk to a simmer. Pour the hot nut milk over the chocolate chips and allow to sit for a couple of minutes. Mix until smooth using a rubber spatula. Allow to cool for 5 minutes, then pour the ganache over the cooled cake and allow to set. Cover and store in the refrigerator for up to 3 days.

TIP: The touch of espresso powder in this cake enhances the natural flavor of the cocoa powder. Additionally, using boiling water helps bloom both the cocoa powder and espresso powder for an intense chocolate flavor.

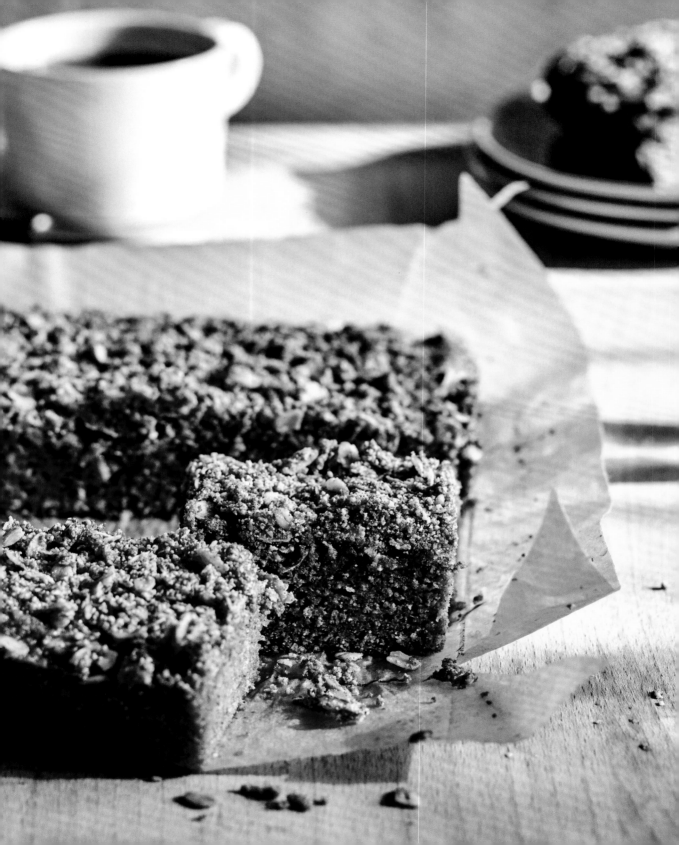

Cinnamon Crumb Coffee Cake

PREP TIME// 15 minutes

COOK TIME// 35 minutes

SERVES// 6 to 8

Topping

½ cup almond flour

½ cup old-fashioned rolled oats

¼ cup coconut sugar

¼ cup coconut oil, chilled

1¼ teaspoons ground cinnamon

¼ teaspoon ground nutmeg

Pinch of sea salt

Cake

Coconut oil cooking spray, for greasing

1 cup almond flour

¾ cup oat flour

1 teaspoon ground cinnamon

½ teaspoon baking soda

½ teaspoon sea salt

¼ cup coconut oil, melted

2 large eggs, lightly beaten

½ cup full-fat coconut milk, well shaken

⅓ cup pure maple syrup

2 teaspoons vanilla extract

This coffee cake is one of my family's top picks, and it's a must for any family gathering. My recipe is inspired by the box cinnamon coffee cake my mom used to always make for Passover. The topping is crumbly with a nice hint of cinnamon, and the base of the cake is fluffy and lightly sweetened. In the summer, I add fresh blueberries to the cake for a burst of fruit flavor.

1   **For the Topping:** In a medium bowl, use your hands to mix together the almond flour, oats, coconut sugar, coconut oil, cinnamon, nutmeg, and salt until a crumble begins to form. Place in the refrigerator until ready to use.

2   **For the Cake:** Preheat the oven to 350°F. Line an 8 × 8-inch baking dish with parchment paper, allowing the sides to hang over as handles, and grease with cooking spray.

3   In a large bowl, whisk together the almond flour, oat flour, cinnamon, baking soda, and salt.

4   In a medium bowl, whisk together the coconut oil, eggs, coconut milk, maple syrup, and vanilla.

5   Make a well in the dry mixture and pour the wet mixture into the well. Stir gently until combined. Pour the batter into the prepared baking dish. Sprinkle the crumble topping evenly over the top. Bake on the middle rack for 30 to 35 minutes, until an inserted toothpick comes out clean.

6   Allow to cool in the pan completely. Slice and serve. Store in an airtight container at room temperature for up to 4 days.

TIP: Add 1 cup blueberries to the batter and gently fold them into the batter to coat them in the oat flour.

Carrot Cake

with Cashew Cream Cheese Frosting

PREP TIME // 20 minutes +
15 minutes soaking
COOK TIME // 35 minutes
MAKES // one 9-inch cake

Carrot Cake

Coconut oil cooking spray, for greasing

1½ cups white whole wheat flour

2 tablespoons ground flaxseed

1½ teaspoons ground cinnamon

1½ teaspoons ground ginger

½ teaspoon ground nutmeg

1½ teaspoons baking powder

1 teaspoon baking soda

½ teaspoon sea salt

½ cup pure maple syrup

½ cup unsweetened applesauce

½ cup unsweetened nut milk

¼ cup coconut oil, melted

1¾ cups grated carrots

¼ cup golden raisins

½ cup toasted pecans, chopped

½ cup unsweetened coconut flakes, toasted (see Note on page 76), to garnish

Cashew Cream Cheese Frosting

1 cup raw cashews

Hot water (115°F to 120°F), to cover cashews

3 tablespoons pure maple syrup

2 tablespoons unsweetened nut milk, plus additional as needed

2 teaspoons fresh lemon juice

Pinch of sea salt

This carrot cake was one of the first cakes I sold when I started my plant-based food business in high school. Inspired by the carrot cake from Candle Café in New York City, my twist includes using natural sweeteners and whole grains. The cake base is full of spices, nuts, and freshly grated carrots, giving it the familiar texture everyone loves, but it's not super sweet. Complete with a creamy cashew-based "cream cheese" frosting, this is a showpiece dessert for any celebration.

1 **For the Carrot Cake:** Preheat the oven to 350°F. Grease a 9-inch cake pan with cooking spray.

2 In a large bowl, whisk together the flour, flaxseed, cinnamon, ginger, nutmeg, baking powder, baking soda, and salt.

3 In a medium bowl, whisk together the maple syrup, applesauce, nut milk, coconut oil, and vanilla. Make a well in the flour mixture and add the maple syrup mixture to the center of the well. Stir gently until just combined.

4 Fold in the carrots, raisins, and pecans. Pour the batter into the cake pan and smooth the top. Bake on the middle rack for 28 to 35 minutes, until an inserted toothpick comes out clean. Remove from the oven and allow to cool for 20 minutes in the pan, then place on a wire rack to cool completely.

5 **For the Cashew Cream Cheese Frosting:** In a small heatproof bowl, cover the cashews with hot water and allow to soak for 15 minutes to soften. Drain and discard the liquid.

6 Transfer the softened cashews to the carafe of a high-speed blender and add the maple syrup, nut milk, lemon juice, and salt. Blend until smooth, adding more nut milk if the icing is too thick.

7 Spread the frosting over the top of the cake and garnish with the toasted coconut flakes. Cover and store in the refrigerator for up to 3 days.

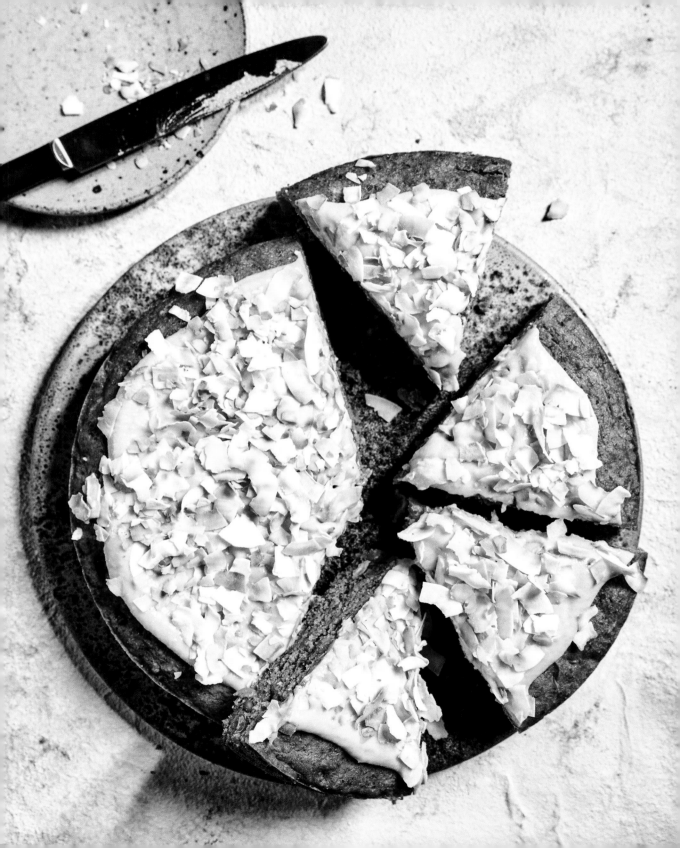

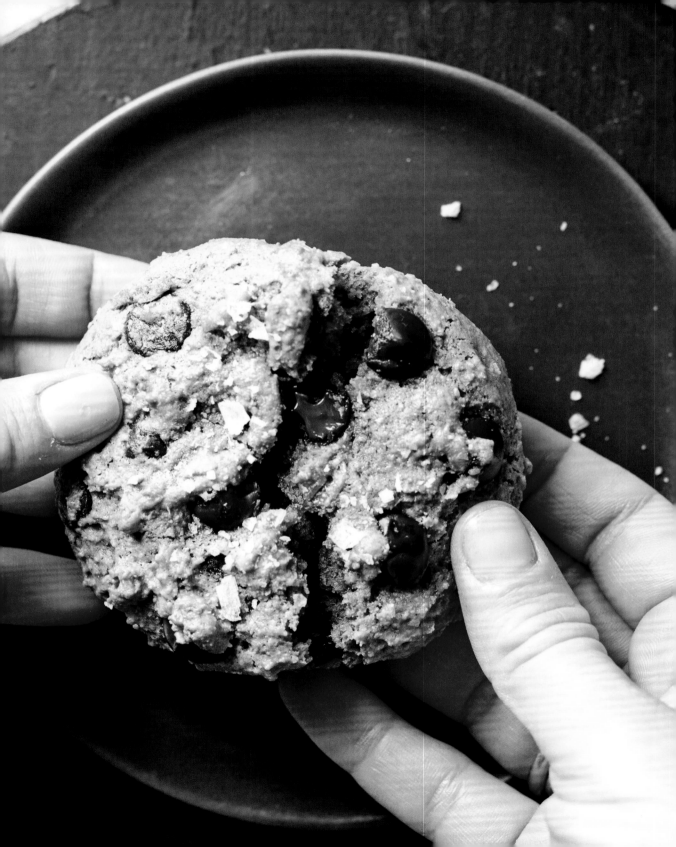

Chocolate Chip Oat Cookies

PREP TIME// 15 minutes
COOK TIME// 12 minutes
MAKES// 16 cookies

1 cup almond flour

1½ cups oat flour

1 teaspoon baking soda

½ teaspoon sea salt

⅓ cup coconut oil, melted

⅔ cup coconut sugar

1 teaspoon vanilla extract

2 large eggs, room temperature, lightly beaten

½ cup old-fashioned rolled oats

1 cup stevia-sweetened dark chocolate chips (I like Lily's)

Flaky sea salt, to garnish

A good chocolate chip cookie recipe is something I always have in my back pocket. They are the ideal last-minute dessert, both quick to make and also so delicious. I use rolled oats as well as flaky sea salt in this version for added texture compared to the classic chocolate chip cookie.

1 Preheat the oven to 350°F. Line two baking sheets with parchment paper.

2 In a large bowl, whisk together the almond flour, oat flour, baking soda, and salt.

3 In a separate large bowl, whisk together the coconut oil, coconut sugar, vanilla, and eggs until creamy and smooth.

4 Make a well in the dry ingredients and add the wet ingredients to the center of the well. Stir until just combined. Add the oats and chocolate chips and fold until incorporated.

5 Scoop the dough using a cookie scoop (or a little less than ¼ cup) onto the prepared baking sheets about 1 inch apart. Press down lightly with your fingers to flatten the tops. Sprinkle with some of the flaky sea salt.

6 Bake on the middle rack for 8 to 12 minutes (depending on how chewy you like your cookies), until golden brown. Allow to cool in the pan for 10 minutes before enjoying. Store in an airtight container for up to 4 days.

Watermelon-Kiwi Ice Pops

PREP TIME// 10 minutes + 8 hours
freezing
MAKES// 6 pops

1½ cups seedless watermelon cubes

1 cup coconut water or water

1 kiwi, peeled and thinly sliced

I always make these fruit-filled ice pops with my nieces and nephews, Frieda, Norman, Salvo, and Jonah, during the summertime. The coconut water hydrates and the fruit adds fiber, perfect for hot days at the beach or just in the backyard.

1 In the carafe of a high-speed blender, blend the watermelon and coconut water until smooth. Divide the kiwi slices among six ice pop molds. Pour in the watermelon mixture. Place ice pop sticks and tops on the mold. Freeze for 8 hours, or until solid.

2 When ready to serve, run the ice pop mold under hot water for a couple of seconds to release the frozen pops.

3 **Fun adult twist:** Use an ice pop instead of an ice cube to chill a tequila or vodka citrus cocktail. The watermelon becomes a surprise added flavor!

TIP: Feel free to use any fresh fruit you have on hand inside the pops. I love berries, mango, and pineapple. Unsweetened coconut flakes are also a nice addition.

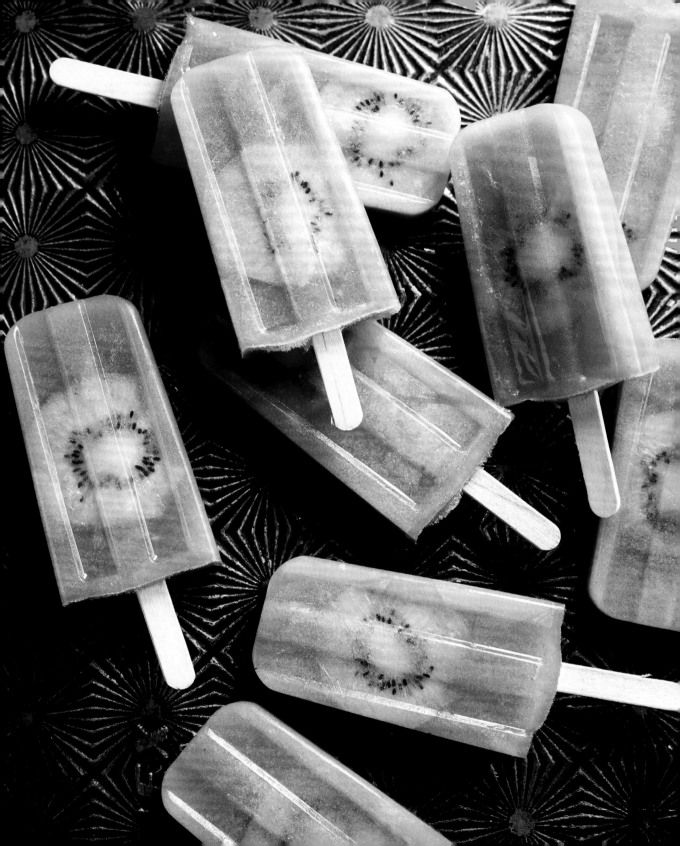

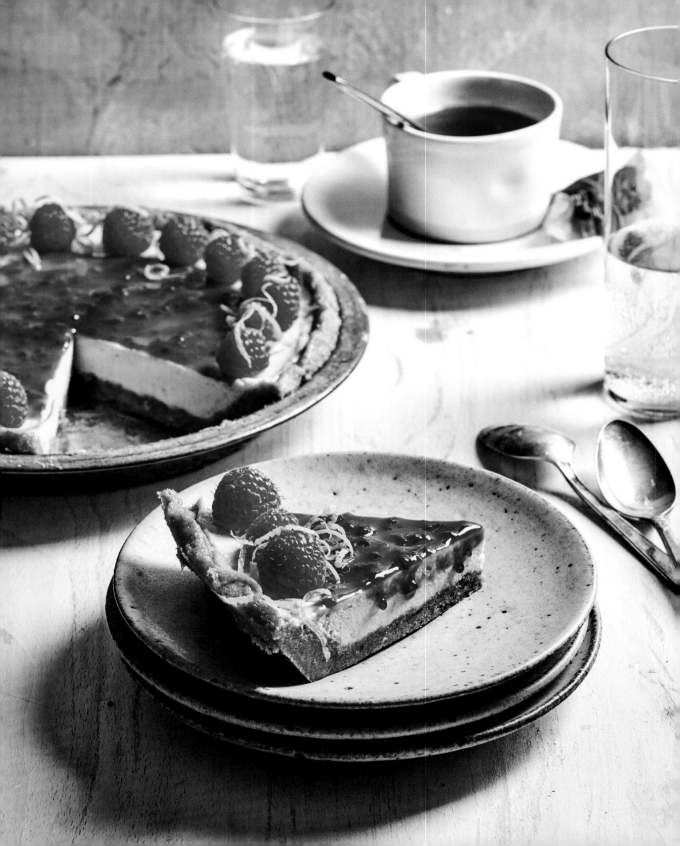

Lemon Raspberry Tart

PREP TIME// 20 minutes +
15 minutes soaking + 4 hours
refrigeration
MAKES// one 9-inch tart

Crust

¾ cup pitted Medjool dates, halved

Hot water (115°F to 120°F), to cover dates

1 cup oat flour

1 cup raw walnuts

2 tablespoons coconut oil, melted

½ teaspoon sea salt

1 tablespoon water (optional)

Filling

1½ cups raw cashews

Hot water (115°F to 120°F), to cover cashews

½ cup unsweetened canned coconut cream

2 tablespoons coconut oil

¼ cup pure maple syrup

1 lemon, zested, plus more to taste

⅓ cup fresh lemon juice, plus more to taste

2 teaspoons vanilla extract

¼ teaspoon sea salt

Topping

⅓ cup fruit-sweetened raspberry jam

1 cup fresh raspberries

½ lemon, zested

Perfect for summer, it's almost as if raspberry lemonade became a pie. Plus, it's entirely vegan and dairy-free. Using blended cashews and coconut cream makes for an easy no-bake filling that is creamy but still light from all the fresh lemon zest and juice.

1 **For the Crust:** In a small heatproof bowl, cover the dates with hot water and allow to soak for 15 minutes to soften. Drain and discard the liquid.

2 In the bowl of a food processor fitted with the blade attachment, pulse the oat flour and walnuts until chopped. Add the softened dates, coconut oil, and salt and puree until a dough forms. Add water, if necessary, to bind. Press evenly into a 9-inch pie plate.

3 **For the Filling:** In a small heatproof bowl, cover the cashews with hot water and allow to soak for 15 minutes to soften. Drain and discard the liquid.

4 Wipe out the food processor. Still using the blade attachment, blend the softened cashews, coconut cream, coconut oil, maple syrup, lemon zest, lemon juice, vanilla, and salt until very smooth. Taste and add more juice and zest if you desire more pucker. Scrape the filling into the tart crust and smooth the top. Cover and refrigerate for 4 hours, or until the center filling is set.

5 **For the Topping:** Spread the raspberry jam in the center of the tart and top with fresh raspberries. Sprinkle with lemon zest and serve. Cover and store in the refrigerator for up to 3 days.

TIP: This is a great make-ahead dessert recipe. It can be stored in the refrigerator for 3 days or in the freezer for up to 1 month. Thaw and add the raspberry topping before serving.

Apple Walnut Crisp

PREP TIME// 20 minutes +
15 minutes soaking
COOK TIME// 50 minutes
SERVES// 6 to 8

Filling

Coconut oil cooking spray, for greasing

5 medium Granny Smith or other tart apples (about 2 pounds), peeled and thinly sliced

1 lemon, juiced

1 teaspoon ground cinnamon

Topping

1 cup pitted Medjool dates, halved

Hot water (115°F to 120°F), to cover dates

1½ cups old-fashioned rolled oats

1½ cups raw walnuts

1 teaspoon vanilla extract

1 teaspoon ground cinnamon

½ teaspoon ground nutmeg

¼ teaspoon sea salt

½ medium Granny Smith apple, peeled, cored, and roughly chopped

3 tablespoons coconut oil, melted, or unsweetened natural almond butter

When fall rolls around and so many different kinds of apples are in season, this is the dessert I immediately crave. I always look for tart apples for this recipe because they have the perfect sweetness after baking. I also like using pureed apple in the topping to help naturally sweeten and bind the crumble. In the summer months, I make this crisp using fresh berries, plums, or peaches. It's truly a dessert for every season.

1 **For the Filling:** Preheat the oven to 350°F. Grease an 11 × 7-inch baking dish with coconut oil spray.

2 In a large bowl, combine the apples, lemon juice, and cinnamon and mix to combine. Pour into the prepared baking dish.

3 **For the Topping:** In a small heatproof bowl, cover the dates with hot water and allow to soak for 15 minutes to soften. Drain and discard the liquid.

4 In the bowl of a food processor fitted with the blade attachment, pulse 1 cup of the oats, 1 cup of the walnuts, the vanilla, cinnamon, nutmeg, and salt until roughly chopped. Add the softened dates, chopped apple, and coconut oil and pulse until combined with a crumbly texture.

5 Add the remaining ½ cup walnuts and ½ cup oats to the crumble in the food processor and pulse until roughly chopped for additional texture in the topping.

6 Sprinkle the topping over the filling and bake on the middle rack, covered with foil, for 30 minutes. Uncover and bake an additional 15 to 20 minutes, until golden brown. Allow to cool for 15 minutes and serve.

TIP: I like to serve this crisp with vegan vanilla ice cream.

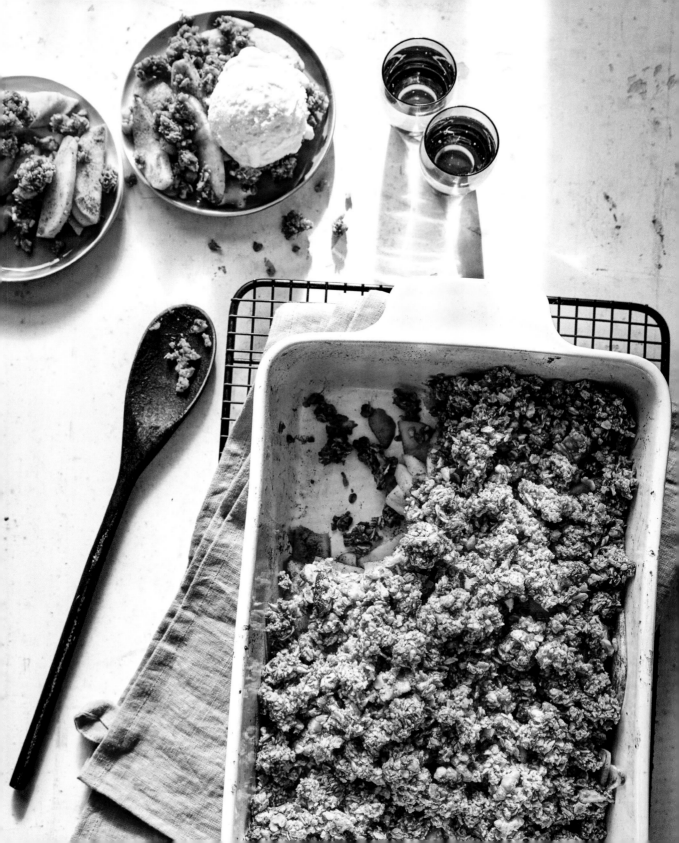

Decadent Ice Cream Cake Four Ways

This ice cream cake recipe has been one of my signature desserts since high school. It's the perfect dessert for a celebration or to bring to a dinner party. The special trick to making it dairy-free is using full-fat coconut milk, and I also keep the crust nut-free by using oats. The vanilla ice cream filling is a good base recipe. I can then add in different fruits, nut butters, extracts, and fresh herbs to make various all-natural ice cream flavors. Here, I'm sharing the classic vanilla base plus my top three flavors from over the years.

PREP TIME// 20 minutes + 15 minutes soaking + 5 hours freezing

MAKES// one 9-inch cake

Crust

1 cup pitted Medjool dates, halved

Hot water (115°F to 120°F), to cover dates

3 cups old-fashioned rolled oats

½ teaspoon sea salt

2 tablespoons unsweetened cocoa powder (optional)

3 to 4 tablespoons water

Vanilla (Base Filling)

1 to 1½ cups pitted Medjool dates, halved

Hot water (115°F to 120°F), to cover dates

1 (13.5-ounce) can full-fat coconut milk, well shaken

3 tablespoons coconut oil

2 teaspoons vanilla extract

Chocolate Peanut Butter

Vanilla (Base Filling)

⅓ cup unsweetened natural creamy peanut butter

2 tablespoons unsweetened cocoa powder

Strawberry

Vanilla (Base Filling)

1¼ cups strawberries, hulled and roughly chopped

Mint Chocolate Chip

Vanilla (Base Filling)

1 cup baby spinach

⅓ to ½ cup fresh mint

½ cup stevia-sweetened dark chocolate chips (I like Lily's)

Optional Chocolate Topping

3 tablespoons unsweetened cocoa power

2 tablespoons coconut oil, melted

3 tablespoons cacao nibs, to garnish

1 **For the Crust:** In a small heatproof bowl, cover the dates with hot water and allow to soak for 15 minutes to soften. Drain and discard the liquid.

2 In the bowl of a food processor fitted with the blade attachment, pulse the oats until almost finely ground. Add the softened dates, salt, and cocoa powder, if desired, and pulse until the mixture comes together to form a dough. Add water by the tablespoon as needed to help the dough come together.

3 Press the crust into the bottom of a 9-inch springform pan.

4 **For the Vanilla (Base Filling):** In a small heatproof bowl, cover 1½ cups dates with hot water and allow to soak for 15 minutes to soften. Drain and discard the liquid.

5 Wipe out the food processor. Still using the blade attachment, puree the softened dates until smooth. Set aside ½ cup of the pureed dates. Add the coconut milk, coconut oil, vanilla, and other desired ingredients for alternative flavors and blend. Taste the filling and adjust the sweetness by adding the reserved pureed dates, if desired.

6 Pour the filling into the springform pan and smooth the top. Sprinkle over any chocolate chips, if using. Place in the freezer for 4 hours, or until completely frozen and set.

7 **For the Optional Chocolate Topping:** If you wish to make the chocolate topping, allow the cake to freeze for just 1 hour.

8 In a small bowl, whisk together the cocoa powder and coconut oil until smooth. Remove the cake from the freezer and drizzle with the chocolate topping (the coconut oil will immediately solidify when it makes contact with the frozen cake). Sprinkle with cacao nibs and place back in the freezer for an additional 3 hours, or until completely frozen and set.

9 Before serving, allow the cake to thaw for 5 to 10 minutes, slice, and serve.

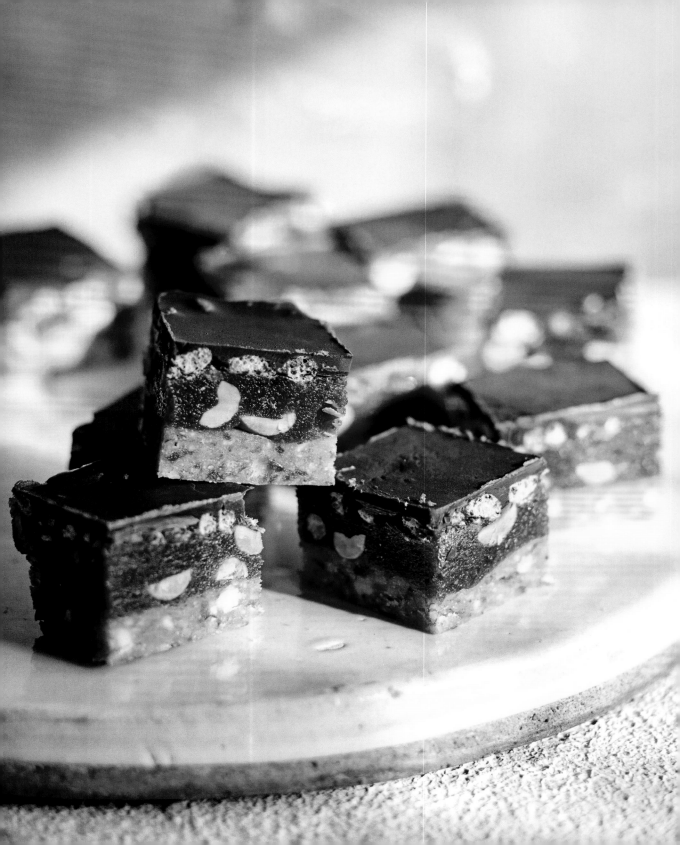

Almost Raw Chocolate Candy Bar

PREP TIME// 30 minutes +
15 minutes soaking + 30 minutes
freezing + 8 hours freezing or
overnight
MAKES// 16 bites

Bottom

½ cup pitted Medjool dates, halved

Hot water (115°F to 120°F), to cover
dates

½ cup raw almonds

1 cup almond flour

½ teaspoon sea salt

2 tablespoons water

Date Caramel Filling

1 cup pitted Medjool dates, halved

Hot water (115°F to 120°F), to cover
dates

½ cup unsweetened natural almond
butter

1 teaspoon vanilla extract

½ teaspoon sea salt

½ cup roasted unsalted peanuts

¼ cup brown rice puffed cereal
(optional)

Topping

¼ cup unsweetened cocoa powder

3 tablespoons coconut oil, melted

Flaky sea salt (optional)

Having a bite-size treat, like these candy bars, in the freezer is a little trick for when you're craving something sweet. They are filled with almonds and peanuts and naturally sweetened using dates. Better yet, they are no-bake, so assembly is even easier.

1 **For the Bottom:** Line a 9 × 5-inch loaf pan with parchment paper. In a small heatproof bowl, cover the dates with hot water and allow to soak for 15 minutes to soften. Drain and discard the liquid.

2 In the bowl of a food processor fitted with the blade attachment, pulse the almonds, flour, and salt until finely chopped. Add the softened dates and continue pulsing until smooth and combined. Add water, a little at a time, if needed, until the date mixture forms a dough.

3 Press the mixture into the bottom of the prepared loaf pan until smooth and even.

4 **For the Date Caramel Filling:** Again, in a small heatproof bowl, cover the dates with hot water and allow to soak for 15 minutes to soften. Drain and discard the liquid.

5 Wipe out the food processor. Still using the blade attachment, pulse the dates, almond butter, vanilla, and salt until smooth and combined. Remove the blade and stir in the peanuts. Spread the mixture evenly over the bottom layer. Sprinkle with the puffed rice cereal, if desired, and press lightly to stick it to the filling. Place in the freezer and allow to freeze for 30 minutes.

6 **For the Topping:** In a small bowl, whisk together the cocoa powder and coconut oil until smooth. Quickly pour over the filling and smooth evenly to cover (coconut oil will immediately solidify when it comes into contact with the cold date caramel filling). Sprinkle with flaky sea salt, if desired. Freeze again for 8 hours or overnight, until set and firm.

7 Remove the solid candy bar from the freezer and cut into 1½ x 1-inch bars. Store in an airtight container in the freezer for up to 1 month.

TIP: Experiment with your favorite nut butter and nuts in this candy bar. The puffed rice cereal, while optional, adds another element of texture.

Brianne Eaton's Peanut Butter Parfait Bars

ATHLETE RECIPE: Brianne Eaton is a heptathlon Olympic bronze medalist turned holistic nutritionist. She has a passion for helping people get to the root cause of their health-related concerns and reverse and prevent them through healthy lifestyle changes. She and her husband, Ashton, an Olympic gold medalist, live in Portland, Oregon, with their son, Ander, and dog, Zora.

"These bars are inspired by one of my favorite ice cream treats from Dairy Queen, the Peanut Buster Parfait. The funny backstory to this recipe is that there was a week a few years ago when I had a craving for one of these delicious treats every night of that week. The craving was so strong I knew I had to develop a homemade version made with whole, nutritious ingredients. My Peanut Butter Parfait Bars are made with coconut milk and cashews and are also dairy-free, gluten-free, and vegan. They are the perfect sweet treat that satisfies all my late-night cravings."

1 For the Crust: Line an 8 × 8-inch baking dish with parchment paper.

2 In the bowl of a food processor fitted with the blade attachment, pulse the almonds until finely ground and almond meal forms. Add the coconut flakes, dates, coconut oil, salt, and water and pulse again until well combined and a dough forms.

3 Press the crust into the bottom of the prepared baking dish and evenly spread. Place in the freezer to chill while you prepare the filling.

4 For the Caramel Sauce: Wipe out the food processor. Still using the blade attachment, blend the dates, salt, vanilla, coconut oil, and water until smooth and creamy. Transfer to a small bowl and set aside. Wipe out the food processor one more time.

5 For the Ice Cream: In a small heatproof bowl, cover the cashews with hot water, and allow to soak for 1 hour. Drain and discard the liquid.

6 Transfer the softened cashews to the food processor and add the coconut milk, coconut oil, maple syrup, salt, and vanilla. Blend until very smooth and creamy.

recipe continues

PREP TIME// 35 minutes + 1 hour soaking + 5 hours 30 minutes
MAKES// 16 bars

Crust

1½ cups raw almonds

¼ cup unsweetened coconut flakes

½ cup pitted Medjool dates

1 tablespoon coconut oil

Pinch of sea salt

2 teaspoons water

Caramel Sauce

1 cup pitted Medjool dates

¼ teaspoon sea salt

½ teaspoon vanilla extract

1 tablespoon coconut oil, melted

½ cup water

Ice Cream

1 cup raw cashews

Hot water (115°F to 120°F), to cover cashews

1 (13.5-ounce) can full-fat coconut milk, well shaken

3 tablespoons coconut oil, melted

⅓ cup pure maple syrup

Pinch of sea salt

1½ teaspoons vanilla extract

¼ cup unsweetened natural peanut butter

¼ cup roasted and salted peanuts

Chocolate Topping

2 ounces 100% cacao chocolate (I like Baker's), chopped

1 tablespoon coconut oil

Flaky sea salt, to garnish

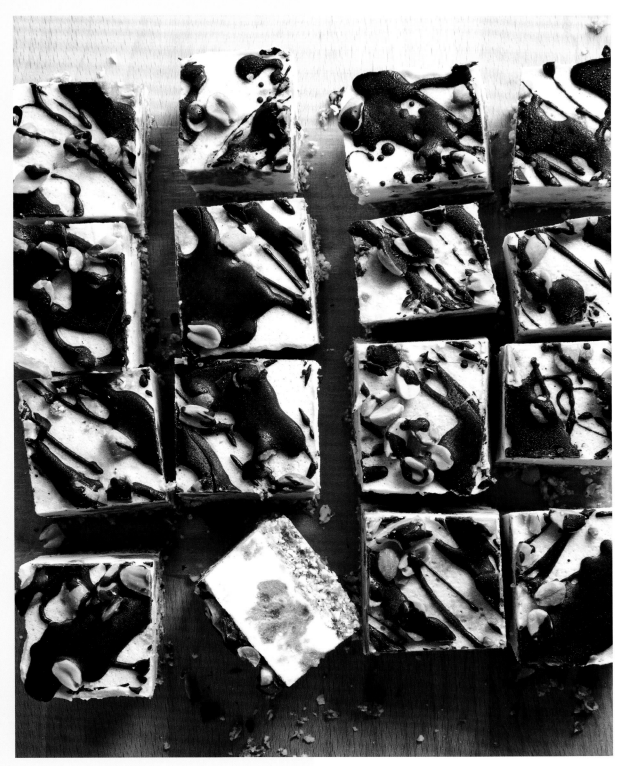

7 To Assemble: Remove the crust from the freezer and pour the ice cream base evenly over the crust. Using a toothpick, add dabs of caramel sauce and peanut butter. Then swirl the dabs with the toothpick throughout the layer of ice cream to make a marble design.

8 Sprinkle peanuts over the top and place in the freezer for 30 minutes to set slightly before drizzling the topping.

9 For the Chocolate Topping: Fill a small pot with 1 inch of water and bring to a simmer. Place the chocolate and coconut oil in a small glass or heatproof bowl and place the bowl over the pot with the simmering water. Allow the chocolate to melt, stirring frequently to combine. (You can also microwave in 15-second intervals, stirring throughout, until completely melted.)

10 Once the ice cream has set, drizzle the chocolate topping over the top and sprinkle with flaky sea salt. Place back in the freezer for 4 hours, or until frozen completely.

11 When ready to serve, allow to sit at room temperature for 10 minutes before cutting into bars.

Ajee' Wilson's Cinnamon Chips
with Fruit Salsa

ATHLETE RECIPE: Ajee' Wilson is a New Jersey native who moved to Philadelphia after graduating high school to pursue a professional career in track and field. She specializes in the 800 meter and is the American record holder in the event, both indoors and outdoors. Other career accomplishments include simultaneously earning a bachelor of science degree at Temple University, competing in the 2016 and 2021 Olympics, and winning eleven national titles.

"Anyone who knows me can attest to how much I *love* sweets and treats. I'm talking about those feel-good snacks and meals that make you do a little dance in anticipation! As we've all heard time and time again, everything in moderation! So, when I've got a little sweet tooth and want to make a healthier choice, this recipe is one of my go-tos! This recipe is inspired by one of my mom's signature sweet treats—whenever I go home, this is always on the table."

1 **For the Cinnamon Chips:** Preheat the oven to 350°F. Line a baking sheet with parchment paper.

2 In a small bowl, combine the coconut sugar, cinnamon, and salt. Place the tortilla wedges onto the prepared baking sheet and lightly spray with cooking spray. Sprinkle with the cinnamon sugar. Bake on the middle rack for 10 to 13 minutes, rotating the baking sheet halfway through cooking.

3 **For the Fruit Salsa:** In a medium bowl, combine the apples, strawberries, kiwis, lemon zest, lemon juice, and coconut sugar. Serve with the cinnamon chips.

PREP TIME// 15 minutes
COOK TIME// 13 minutes
SERVES// 4

Cinnamon Chips

⅓ cup coconut sugar

2 teaspoons ground cinnamon

Pinch of sea salt

6 (8-inch) brown rice tortillas, cut into 8 wedges

Coconut oil cooking spray

Fruit Salsa

2 Granny Smith apples, peeled and diced small

2 cups strawberries, hulled and diced small

2 kiwis, peeled and diced small

½ lemon, zested

3 tablespoons fresh lemon juice

1 tablespoon coconut sugar

Condiments/ Dressings

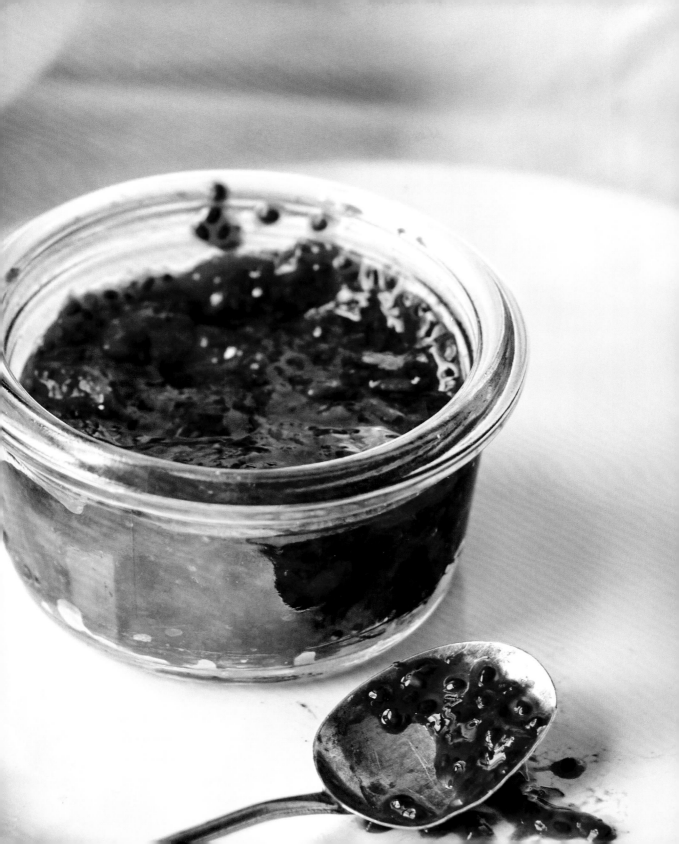

This chapter highlights all the different dressings, sauces, spreads, and finishing touches that I use throughout the book. These sauces are *so* versatile; try adding them to any simple meal or to other recipes within the book! I think plant-based sauces are fun to develop—I often use blended nuts to make a creamy base and then play with different spices and fresh herbs for a powerful flavor that is sure to jazz up any recipe. I try to make a couple of these condiments at the beginning of the week to have in the fridge. It really helps with meal prep and makes even the plainest roasted veggies delicious during weeks when I don't have much time for cooking. The Almond Parmesan (page 241) is always a crowd-pleaser for pretty much any pasta or roasted vegetable dish. The Quick-Pickled Red Onions (page 238) can be added to almost any bowl or salad, and the Roasted Tomato Sauce (page 236) is a freezer staple for an impressive meal on the fly.

Roasted Tomato Sauce

PREP TIME// 5 minutes

COOK TIME// 35 minutes

MAKES// 1 cup

4 cups cherry tomatoes

1 small yellow onion, thinly sliced

3 garlic cloves, sliced

4 sprigs fresh thyme

3 tablespoons avocado oil

Sea salt and freshly ground black pepper to taste

This recipe creates a delicious tomato sauce all year long. Roasting the tomatoes and onions brings out their natural sugars, producing a rustic tomato sauce you will want to put on everything. It's a one-sheet pan sauce that allows the tomatoes, garlic, and onions to caramelize for a hint of veggie sweetness. It's also perfect any time of year because the roasting really helps bring out the flavor of the cherry tomatoes, no matter the ripeness.

1 Preheat the oven to 400°F. Line a rimmed baking sheet with parchment paper.

2 In a large bowl, toss the tomatoes, onion, garlic, and thyme with avocado oil. Season with salt and pepper.

3 Place the mixture on the prepared baking sheet and roast on the middle rack for 25 to 30 minutes, until tomatoes are lightly golden and broken down.

4 Remove the thyme sprigs and discard. Transfer the roasted vegetables to the carafe of a high-speed blender and blend until smooth. Season with additional salt and pepper, if necessary.

5 Use right away or store in an airtight container in the refrigerator for up to 5 days or in the freezer for up to 1 month.

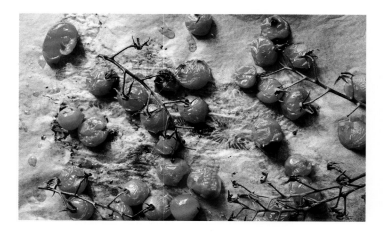

TRY THIS recipe in the Quinoa Crust Pizza with Broccoli Rabe and Almond Ricotta (page 135).

Vegan Ranch Dressing

PREP TIME// 10 minutes + 20 minutes soaking

MAKES// 1 cup

1 cup raw cashews

Hot water (115°F to 120°F), to cover cashews, plus additional ¾ cup

1 garlic clove

2 tablespoons extra-virgin olive oil

3 tablespoons fresh lemon juice

2 teaspoons apple cider vinegar

1 teaspoon onion powder

½ teaspoon ground mustard or Dijon mustard

2 tablespoons chopped fresh dill or 1 tablespoon dried dill

1 tablespoon chopped fresh chives

Pinch of sweet paprika

Sea salt and freshly ground black pepper to taste

Ranch is a condiment I never really found myself missing as a vegan until I made this vegan ranch sauce that uses fresh dill and chives—it's a touch of herby flavor that highlights all the other flavors in a recipe. Use on a salad, grain bowl, and roasted veggies or as the sauce in a wrap. Blending cashews for the dressing base is key to the smooth texture and also gives you a boost of heart-healthy fats.

1   In a small heatproof bowl, cover the cashews with hot water and allow to soak for 20 minutes to soften. Drain and discard the liquid.

2   Transfer the softened cashews to the carafe of a high-speed blender and add the garlic, ¾ cup hot water, olive oil, lemon juice, vinegar, onion powder, mustard, dill, chives, and paprika. Blend until smooth. Season with salt and pepper to taste.

3   Store in an airtight container in the refrigerator for up to 1 week.

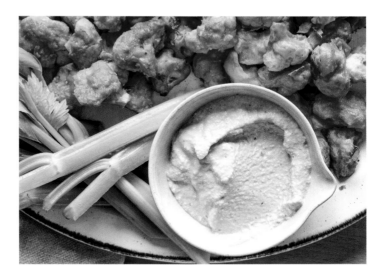

TRY THIS recipe with the Buffalo Cauliflower Wings (page 165) and the BBQ Fajita Bowl (page 89).

Quick-Pickled Red Onions

PREP TIME// 5 minutes + cooling
to room temperature
COOK TIME// 5 minutes
MAKES// 1 cup

1 medium red onion, thinly sliced

2 garlic cloves, sliced

1 teaspoon black peppercorns

⅔ cup rice wine vinegar

2 teaspoons sea salt

These pickled red onions are the ideal addition to almost any recipe. I love adding them to eggs as well as avocado toast. They add a light tang and are easy to make. The quick-pickling liquid in this recipe is just heated salt and rice wine vinegar with spices, which softens the vegetables and brings out their natural sweetness. Try using some other veggies like carrots, cucumbers, and peppers.

1 Place the onion, garlic, and peppercorns in a small mason jar or heatproof container with a lid. Set aside.

2 In a small saucepan over medium heat, simmer the vinegar and salt until the salt dissolves, about 2 minutes. Pour the vinegar mixture over the onion slices and allow to cool to room temperature, about 20 minutes. Cover tightly and store in the refrigerator for up to 2 weeks.

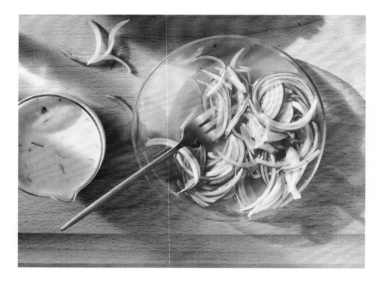

TIP: You can use any type of vinegar here. I like rice vinegar because its flavor is less acidic than many other vinegars. If you prefer a stronger-flavored vinegar, add equal parts water to the heated liquid before pouring over the vegetables.

TRY THIS recipe with the Falafel Slider Greek Salad Bowl (page 105).

Lemon Tahini Dressing

PREP TIME// 5 minutes

MAKES// 1 cup

½ cup tahini, well stirred

½ cup plus 1 tablespoon fresh lemon juice

¼ cup extra-virgin olive oil

½ cup hot water (115°F to 120°F)

2 tablespoons chopped fresh flat-leaf parsley

Sea salt to taste

Tahini is a nutty paste made from grinding sesame seeds and it's one of my most used ingredients. I grew up eating tahini from an early age thanks to my Turkish roots and my mom's recipes. This is a dressing I always have in my refrigerator. It's the perfect finishing touch for not only salads but also roasted veggies and grain bowls.

In a medium bowl, whisk together tahini, lemon juice, olive oil, and hot water until smooth (the tahini may seize at first, just continue whisking for 30 seconds, or until smooth). Add parsley, season with salt, and stir to combine. Use immediately or store in an airtight container in the refrigerator for up to 1 week.

Superfood Mixed-Berry Chia Jam

PREP TIME// 5 minutes

COOK TIME// 20 minutes

MAKES// 1½ cups

2 cups fresh or frozen mixed berries (raspberries, blackberries, blueberries, or strawberries)

½ lemon, zested

3 tablespoons fresh lemon juice

1 navel orange, zested and juiced

¼ cup chia seeds

½ cup water

This jam is a staple condiment in my kitchen. Not only is it sweetened naturally with berries and citrus juice instead of added sugar, but it's also naturally thickened with chia seeds instead of pectin. Chia seeds come from a plant related to mint and provide you with a lot of natural energy, fiber, and antioxidants. They have so much nutritional value to offer, and they are quite filling. This is a jam that's perfect for spreading on toast; it can also be used in place of the raspberry jam in my Lemon Raspberry Tart (page 221).

1 In a small saucepan, combine the berries, lemon zest, lemon juice, orange zest, orange juice, and chia seeds. Add the water and bring to a boil. Reduce the heat and allow to simmer for 20 minutes, stirring frequently.

2 Remove from the heat and mash the fruit with a potato masher or wooden spoon. Allow to cool for 20 minutes, or until the mixture is thickened. Store in an airtight container in the refrigerator for up to 1 week.

TRY THIS recipe with the Almond Berry Overnight Oats (page 38).

Almond Parmesan

PREP TIME// 5 minutes

MAKES// ½ cup

½ cup raw almonds

½ teaspoon sea salt

2 tablespoons nutritional yeast

½ teaspoon garlic powder

This almond "parm" is my substitute to make any cheese recipe dairy-free. It adds a nutty flavor from the almonds as well as a little bit of additional protein. The cheese flavor is thanks to the nutritional yeast, which also adds protein, B vitamins, and trace minerals, like zinc. Sprinkle on eggs in the morning, or add to a creamy salad dressing to make it richer (like my Vegan Caesar Dressing on page 90).

1   In a high-speed blender or mini food processor, pulse all the ingredients until finely ground. It should have a consistency like ground Parmesan cheese.

2   Store in an airtight container for up to 2 weeks.

TRY THIS recipe with the Vegan Chickpea Kale Caesar (page 90), Supergreen Pasta (page 112), or the Pesto Farro Risotto with Snap Peas and Asparagus (page 140).

Almond Ricotta

PREP TIME// 5 minutes + 2 hours refrigeration

MAKES// 2 cups

2 cups blanched almonds or raw cashews

¼ cup nutritional yeast

3 tablespoons fresh lemon juice

⅔ cup hot water (115°F to 120°F)

⅓ cup unsweetened nut milk

¼ teaspoon garlic powder

½ teaspoon sea salt

This nut-based dairy-free "ricotta" is creamy and light and adds a flavor boost to almost any sweet or savory recipe. One of my favorite ways to eat it is to spread it on a piece of warm whole wheat sourdough toast and drizzle with Superfood Mixed-Berry Chia Jam (page 240).

In the carafe of a high-speed blender, blend all the ingredients until a ricotta-like texture forms. Chill for 2 hours before using. Store in the refrigerator in an airtight container for up to 4 days.

TRY THIS recipe with the Quinoa Crust Pizza with Broccoli Rabe and Almond Ricotta (page 135).

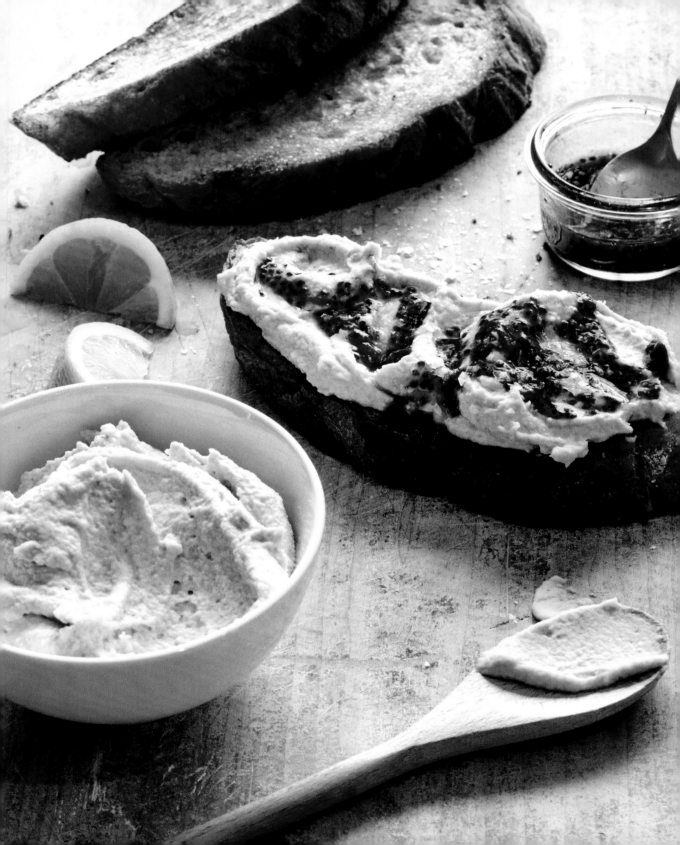

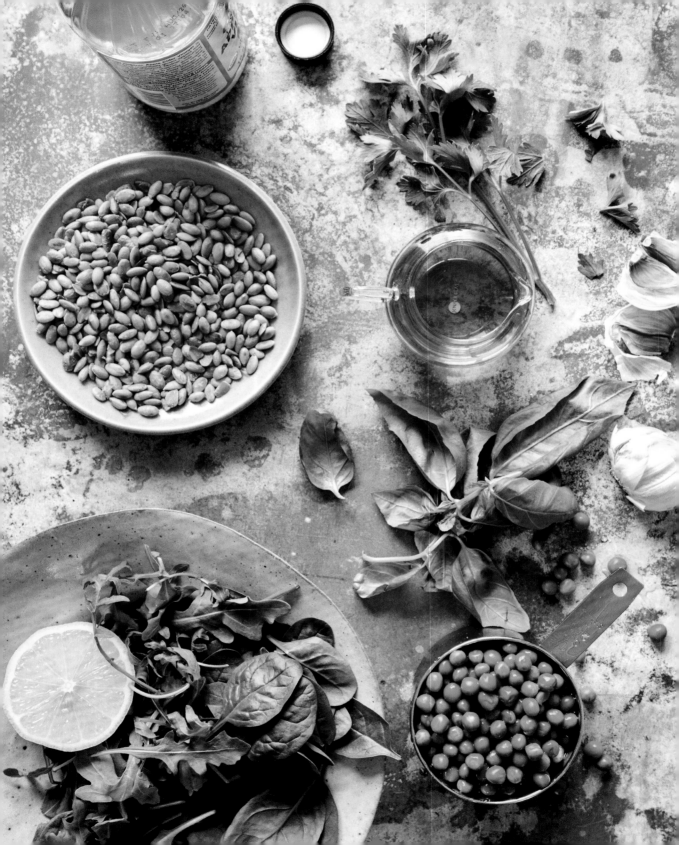

Pea and Pumpkin Seed Pesto

PREP TIME// 5 minutes

MAKES// 1½ cups

1 cup baby spinach

1 cup baby arugula

1 cup frozen peas, thawed for 30 minutes

1 cup packed fresh basil

½ cup fresh flat-leaf parsley

¼ cup roasted pumpkin seeds

2 garlic cloves

6 tablespoons fresh lemon juice

2 tablespoons apple cider vinegar

Sea salt and freshly ground black pepper to taste

¼ cup extra-virgin olive oil

Pesto is my reliable sauce to add to a protein or roasted veggies. Feel free to use any of the greens and herbs in your kitchen. I love using a mix of spinach, arugula, parsley, basil, and kale for all different vitamins and nutrients as well as a rich, healthy flavor. The peas add a creaminess to the pesto and allow you to cut down on too much olive oil. The pumpkin seeds impart a rich, almost nutty flavor to the pesto.

1 In the bowl of a food processor fitted with the blade attachment, pulse the spinach, arugula, peas, basil, parsley, pumpkin seeds, and garlic until finely chopped. Add the lemon juice and vinegar and season with salt and pepper.

2 With the machine running, slowly drizzle in the olive oil. Blend for 20 to 30 seconds, until smooth. Season with additional salt and pepper, if necessary. Use immediately or store in the refrigerator in an airtight container with a piece of plastic wrap touching the surface for up to 4 days.

TIP: I like to freeze half this recipe to have on hand at any time. If you freeze the pesto in ice cube trays and then transfer the frozen cubes to a plastic bag, you will have an individual-sized portion to toss on some hot cooked pasta whenever you need it!

TRY THIS recipe with the Pesto Farro Risotto with Snap Peas and Asparagus (page 140).

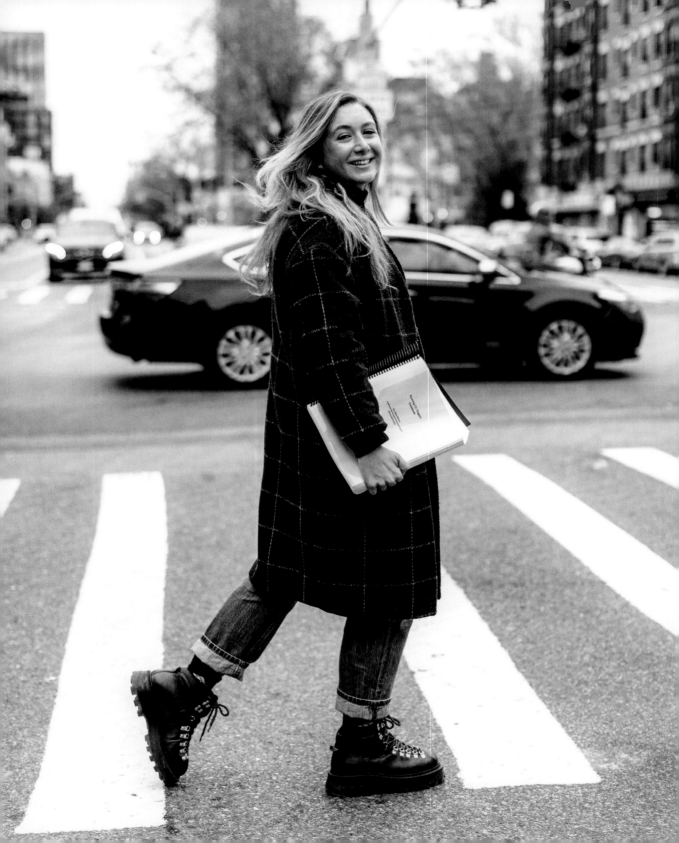

Acknowledgments

Writing this book has been a labor of love and a dream of mine for as long as I can remember. Of course, it wouldn't have been possible without an incredible team of talented, passionate, and hardworking people in my corner, each of whom played a pivotal role in making this book a reality.

I want to thank Penguin Random House and Rodale for the opportunity and platform to publish this book. I am so fortunate for their team of diligent and committed people. Dervla Kelly, my amazing editor, who is just as passionate as I am when it comes to delicious food and everything healthy. Her patience, guidance, and sense of humor through it all has made this process so enjoyable. Jennifer Davis and Lise Sukhu, for the beautiful design and layout of this book. Stephanie Huntwork for the expert art direction during the photo shoot. Lauren Volo, my photographer with the magic eye and meticulous focus. Lauren's team: Monica Pierini, food stylist, and Emma Rowe, her assistant, were so efficient and made everything seem effortless, even though they were working hard in order to cook recipes day after day and style them to perfection. The photoshoot was the highlight of creating this book and I am grateful to all the women who made it happen.

I also want to thank Keith Montero for his incredible photos throughout the years, from capturing me running to events/workshops to in the kitchen cooking—you do it all! Susan Menashe, my aunt and mentor, it is such a special gift to have photos that you took of me as a child displayed in the book. Donalrey Nieva, thank you for the cycling shots throughout the book.

Huge thanks to Laura Arnold, who polished up each recipe and helped bring my vision to fruition. Even during the uncertain times of COVID-19, we were able to work through all the challenges. Laura was instrumental in testing each recipe and making sure the ingredient balance and cooking process for every recipe was foolproof. We worked and cooked together for two months straight and it was inspiring to see someone who works so hard and so passionately, and always with ease and a smile. I also want to thank my friends and family, who continued to recipe-test all summer long as I sent them recipes on a daily basis and then called them, emailed them, and bugged them for feedback. Thank you for the unconditional support—Linda Maleh, Terri Harary, Pauline Shabot, Rachel Harary, Iris Chera, Shiara Robinson.

To my agents, Steve Troha and Jan Baumer at Folio Agency, thank you for believing in me and in this project since day one. Despite the challenges that come with writing a book, you stuck by my side, nudged me patiently, and guided me with your wisdom through all the tough decisions and times of uncertainty. The road was long, but there was no one with whom I would have rather been.

Thank you to Sally Shatzkes, triathlete and mother of five, who has been editing my work since

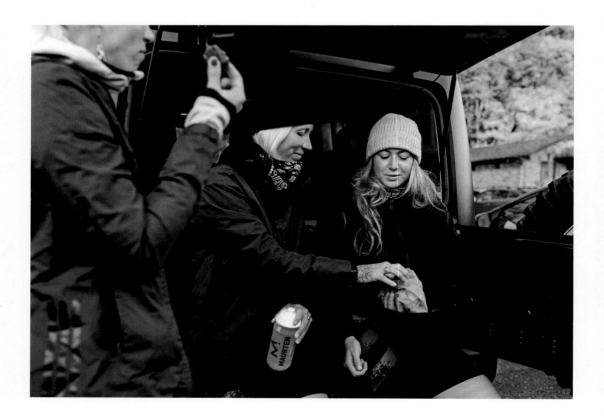

the very beginning of *Running on Veggies*. Her editorial support and all-around inspiration has played a pivotal role in the success of *Running on Veggies*. Thanks to Joseph Benun, who helped me navigate the waters of creating my own brand, and to Jeffrey Dweck, who oversaw all the legal work from our first trademark to some of the biggest contracts of my life.

I owe an enormous amount of gratitude to my family who provide me with love and support. Thank you, Mom, Dad, Pauline, Moey, Rafael, Diana, and Hymie and of course to my beautiful nieces and nephews Frieda, Norman, Salvo, Jonah, Salvo E, and Claudia.

Finally, and most significantly, I would have never written this book without the support of the *Running on Veggies* community. I am continually humbled by the generosity, support, and love that I get from each and every person. Most days I wake up and pinch myself that this is my reality and acknowledge how lucky I am to have this platform to share my story, my passions, my recipes, and my knowledge. It is a blessing that I will never take for granted. When things got tough, I drew motivation from my community and the ways in which I have been able to impact people's lives. Thank you for inspiring me to push toward the finish line so I could achieve this tremendous goal.

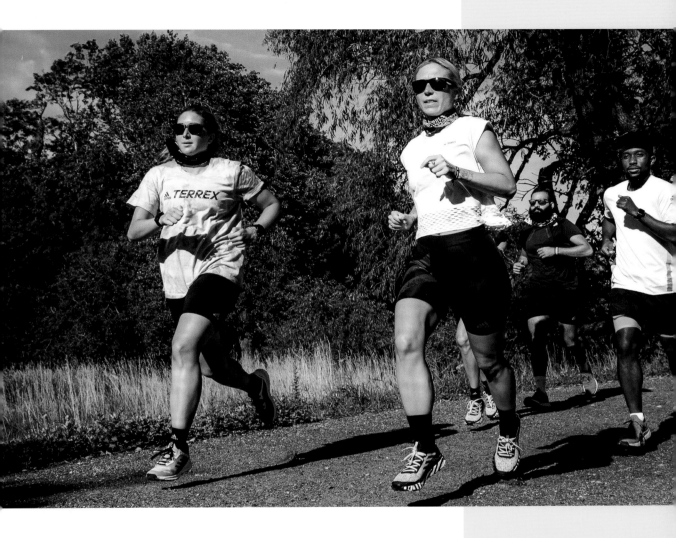
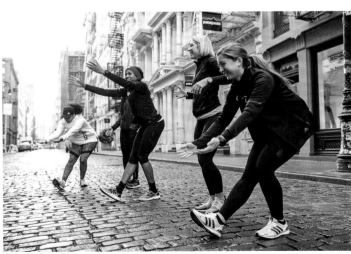

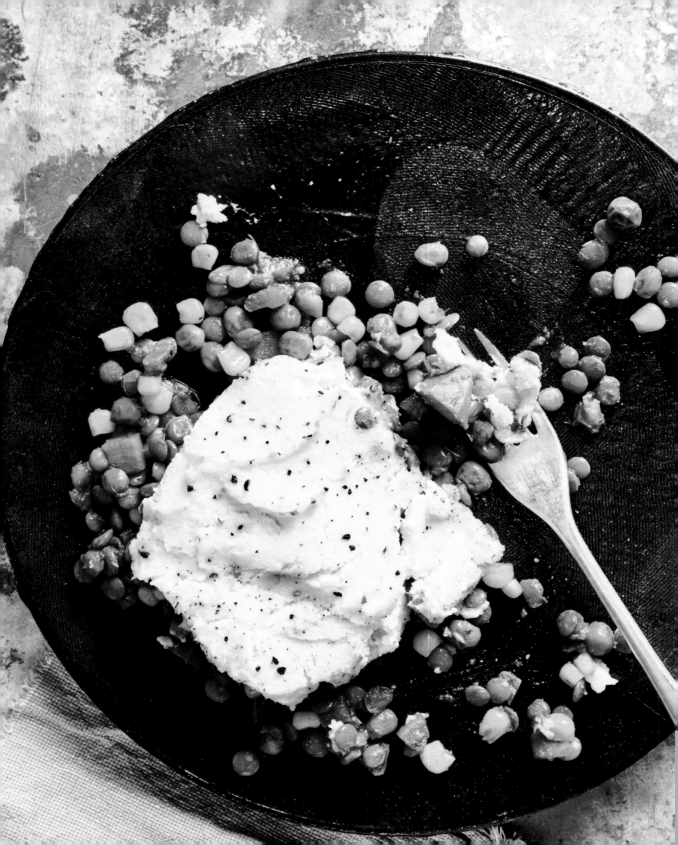

Index